CLINICAL NURSE EDUCATOR COMPETENCIES

CREATING AN EVIDENCE-BASED PRACTICE FOR ACADEMIC CLINICAL NURSE EDUCATORS

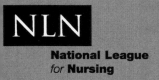

National League
for **Nursing**

CLINICAL NURSE EDUCATOR COMPETENCIES

CREATING AN EVIDENCE-BASED PRACTICE FOR ACADEMIC CLINICAL NURSE EDUCATORS

Edited by:

Teresa Shellenbarger, PhD, RN, CNE, ANEF

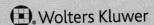

Philadelphia • Baltimore • New York • London
Buenos Aires • Hong Kong • Sydney • Tokyo

Vice President and Publisher: Julie K. Stegman
Executive Editor: Kelley Squazzo
Director of Product Development: Jennifer K. Forestieri
Senior Development Editor: Meredith L. Brittain
Marketing Manager: Katie Schlesinger
Editorial Assistant: Leo Gray
Design Coordinator: Steven Druding
Production Project Manager: Marian Bellus
Manufacturing Coordinator: Karin Duffield
Prepress Vendor: Aptara, Inc.

Shellenbarger, T. (2019). *Clinical Nurse Educator Competencies: Creating an Evidence-Based Practice for Academic Clinical Nurse Educators.* Washington, DC: National League for Nursing.

9 8 7 6 5 4 3

Printed in the United States of America

Library of Congress Cataloging-in-Publication Data

Names: Shellenbarger, Teresa, editor.
Title: Clinical nurse educator competencies : creating an evidence-based practice for academic clinical nurse educators / edited by Teresa Shellenbarger.
Description: Philadelphia : Wolters Kluwer, [2019] | Includes bibliographical references.
Identifiers: LCCN 2018002627 | ISBN 9781975104269 (alk. paper)
Subjects: | MESH: Education, Nursing | Nurse Clinicians–standards | Faculty, Nursing | Clinical Competence | Evidence-Based Nursing
Classification: LCC RT71 | NLM WY 18 | DDC 610.73071/1–dc23
LC record available at https://lccn.loc.gov/2018002627

DRC0818

About the Editor

Teresa Shellenbarger, PhD, RN, CNE, ANEF is Distinguished University Professor and the doctoral program coordinator in the Department of Nursing and Allied Health Professions at Indiana University of Pennsylvania, Indiana, Pennsylvania. She received her bachelor's degree in nursing from the Pennsylvania State University, master of science in nursing from Southern Connecticut State University, and her doctorate in nursing from Widener University.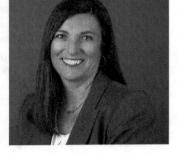

As an experienced nurse educator for more than 25 years, Dr. Shellenbarger has taught a variety of theory and clinical courses at the bachelor, master, and doctoral levels. She has published and presented extensively on topics related to innovative teaching strategies, faculty role development, technology use in nursing education, and clinical nursing education. Co-author of the popular book *Clinical Teaching Strategies in Nursing*, she is a member of the editorial boards for *Nursing Education Perspectives* and *Nurse Educator*, and serves as a reviewer for various other nursing publications.

Dr. Shellenbarger has been active at the National League for Nursing (NLN), having served as a member of the Board of Governors for 6 years. She is currently NLN secretary and participates as a member of various NLN task groups and committees. Additionally, Dr. Shellenbarger is an NLN certified nurse educator and was inducted as an inaugural fellow in the NLN Academy of Nursing Education.

About the Contributors

Wanda Bonnel, PhD, APRN, ANEF is an associate professor at the University of Kansas School of Nursing, Kansas City, Kansas. Dr. Bonnel, a specialist in geriatrics and nursing education, teaches courses in the master and doctoral programs, with ongoing publications and research interests related to clinical education, advanced practice mentoring, and online learning. She is a fellow in the National League for Nursing (NLN) Academy of Nursing Education and recipient of the Chancellor's Distinguished Teaching Award at the University of Kansas. An author of numerous publications in nursing education and geriatrics, Dr. Bonnel has served as a project director for multiple national and teaching grant awards. She is an editorial board member of the *Journal of Gerontological Nursing* and has served as a grant reviewer for the Health Resources and Services Administration and the NLN.

Linda S. Christensen, EdD, JD, RN, CNE is the chief administration officer for the NLN in Washington, DC, a position she has held since 2009. She has more than 35 years of experience in nursing education, with expertise in nursing educator competencies, nursing education, curriculum, and evaluation. She has taught both graduate and undergraduate nursing, as well as online education courses. Additionally, she is an attorney with 20 years of experience of combining nursing and the law. She is frequently a guest speaker on legal issues in nursing education and has authored chapters on nursing law for various books on nursing education.

Melora D. Ferren, MSN, RN-BC is the executive director for discovery and contemporary nursing practice at Indiana University Health, a health care system of 16 facilities. Her nursing career spans 23 years with a clinical background in the emergency department, critical care transport, and leadership. She earned a master's degree in nursing education in 2009, with graduate work including qualitative research on preceptor support and development. She has presented nationally and internationally on leadership and nursing education. Ms. Ferren served as a consultant for the NLN on the *Acceleration to Practice* project and is a social media coordinator for the *Journal of Nursing Administration (JONA)*. She is board certified in nursing professional development and a member of the American Organization of Nurse Executives (AONE), Association for Nursing Professional Development (ANPD), and Sigma Theta Tau.

Erin Killingsworth, PhD, RN, CNE is a clinical assistant professor and program evaluation and accreditation coordinator at the Louise Herrington School of Nursing at Baylor University in Dallas, Texas. Her scholarly work focuses on student and program evaluation, instrument development and validation, and simulation-based learning experiences. Dr. Killingsworth serves as a nurse planner for the International Nursing Association for Clinical Simulation and Learning (INACSL). She has been a nurse educator for more than 10 years and has taught prelicensure, master, and doctoral nursing students.

John D. Lundeen, EdD, RN, CNE, COI is an associate professor and nurse anesthesia simulation coordinator at Samford University in Birmingham, Alabama, where he has taught in the BSN, MSN, and DNP programs for 10 years. His clinical experience consists of medical/surgical and intensive care nursing. Dr. Lundeen has expertise in faculty development, curriculum development and evaluation, test item construction and analysis, and certification. He is active in the NLN, where he currently serves as a member of the Board of Governors. He previously served on the CNE Certification Commission and as the chair of the CNE Test Development Committee and several CNE exam item-writing teams. He has published and presented in the area of faculty peer evaluation and nurse educator certification. Dr. Lundeen is credentialed as a certified nurse educator and certified online instructor.

Amber M. Patrick, PhD, RN, CNE, COI is a cardiac intensive care nurse at Princeton Baptist Medical Center in Birmingham, Alabama, and is currently completing a master's nurse practitioner degree in adult-gerontology acute care. Her clinical education interests include the orientation and integration of new graduate nurses to full-time bedside nursing, full-time bedside nurses to adjunct clinical education, and the continuing education of bedside nurses. She is a former assistant professor in the Ida Moffett School of Nursing, Samford University in Birmingham, Alabama, where she served as full-time undergraduate faculty from 2013 to 2017. She continues to serve as a clinical adjunct for the Ida Moffett School of Nursing. She is also a member of several professional organizations, including Sigma Theta Tau International Honor Society of Nursing (Gamma Eta Chapter), the American Association of Critical-Care Nurses (AACN), and the Alabama and National League for Nursing.

Larry E. Simmons, PhD, RN, CNE, NEA-BC is the director of the Academic Nurse Educator Certification Program (CNE) at the NLN. He has 16 years of experience in testing and certification management and has remained active in faculty roles as adjunct and full-time faculty. He currently teaches in the DNP program at South University Tampa. He received a certificate as a certification specialist from the Institute for Credentialing Excellence (ICE).

Foreword

The National League for Nursing (NLN) continues to lead initiatives focused on the advancement of nursing and nurse educators. This visionary book builds on historical initiatives to recognize the specialized knowledge, skills, and attitudes of the nurse educator to further define the specialty practice role of the clinical nurse educator. Through a rigorous and collaborative process, a specialized task force consisting of NLN leaders and clinical experts from a variety of geographic locations and program types thoroughly reviewed the literature and examined practice analysis data and expert reviews. The result is the development of core competencies and task statements unique to the clinical nurse educator. This publication can serve as a framework to guide excellence in clinical nursing instruction.

The task force used a systematic and iterative process to identify core concepts and develop core competencies and associated task statements. Results were further validated through public comment, thematic evaluation, and confirmatory analysis. This synthesis and validation of academic clinical nurse educator competencies defines a scope of practice for the role of the academic clinical nurse educator. The results provide a standard of excellence central to the performance expectations associated with this specialized role.

Nursing programs may choose to integrate these competencies into graduate nurse educator programs and use them to guide faculty development, establish faculty performance criteria, and develop clinical educator orientation programs. Nursing education commends the diligent efforts of the task force to create core academic clinical nurse educator competencies and task statements. These efforts continue to support the core mission and values of the NLN to promote excellence in nursing and nursing education.

Kathleen A. Poindexter, PhD, RN, CNE
Associate Professor and Assistant Dean of
Undergraduate Programs
Michigan State University College of Nursing
East Lansing, MI
Chair, NLN Academic Nurse Educator
Certification Program Commission

Preface

Clinical nurse educators fill a critical need in nursing education, guiding nursing students as they acquire the knowledge, skills, and attitudes needed to deliver appropriate patient care in a safe and effective way. The work that clinical nurse educators do to prepare competent practitioners is crucial to the future of health care. However, clinical nurse educators must manage this complex work while considering student, health care, and academic factors.

Up to this point, there has not been a guide or set of standards to direct the clinical nurse educator in this advanced area of specialty practice. Even though there is some overlap with the 2012 National League for Nursing (NLN) *Scope of Practice for Academic Nurse Educators*, there are unique aspects of clinical nursing education that were not adequately addressed in those competencies and task statements. This book represents the work of the NLN Task Group on Clinical Nurse Educators and the attempt to clarify the specialized knowledge of the clinical nurse educator. This book provides a framework for this advanced specialty role. It offers a synthesis of the literature and what is currently known about this topic.

Chapter 1, the introduction, provides a description of the process the task group used to develop the competencies and task statements for clinical nurse educators. Chapters 2 through 7 provide an in-depth analysis of the literature for each of the competencies. Chapter 2 focuses on clinical nurse educators functioning within education and health care environments, which includes functioning in the clinical nurse educator role; operationalizing the curriculum; and abiding by legal requirements, ethical guidelines, agency policies, and guiding frameworks. Chapter 3 addresses facilitation of learning in the health care environment. Demonstrating effective interpersonal communication and collaborative interprofessional relationships is the focus for Chapter 4. Chapter 5 discusses the clinical nurse educator's application of clinical expertise in the health care environment. Chapter 6 examines the facilitation of learner development and socialization. Finally, Chapter 7 focuses on the implementation of effective clinical assessment and evaluation strategies.

Chapters 2 through 7 begin with an introduction to the competency and list the specific task statements for the competency. Then the chapter proceeds with a synthesis of the literature. The focus is on the evidence-based nursing literature, supported by other relevant references. The emergent themes related to each competency are described. After this review, the chapter identifies gaps in the literature and concludes with priorities for future research that can be useful in guiding further work.

These competencies and task statements provide a clear indication of the complex role and unique area of practice of the clinical nurse educator. This book can be used as a framework to direct the work of clinical nurse educators. It can also be helpful in designing orientation, mentoring, or other planning of educational programming to ensure that those practicing in the role of a clinical nurse educator have the specialized knowledge needed for success.

Teresa Shellenbarger, PhD, RN, CNE, ANEF

Acknowledgments

I would like to thank the numerous people who assisted in the completion of this book. First, I offer my appreciation to the National League for Nursing (NLN) leadership team for identifying this important gap in nursing education knowledge and recognizing the significance of this work. Linda Christensen, Larry Simmons, and Elaine Tagliareni have been instrumental in moving the work of the clinical nurse educator competencies forward. The members of the Task Group for Clinical Nurse Educator Competencies shared their critical review and insights about clinical nursing education to arrive at the competencies and task statements that now offer a valuable guide for the work of clinical nurse educators. They have written the chapters that appear in this book, and I offer my thanks for their careful synthesis of the literature. Many NLN members also provided input that helped refine the final competencies and task statements for clinical nurse educators. Their valuable contributions have enhanced this work. Finally, I would like to thank Indiana University of Pennsylvania PhD nursing student Jennifer Chicca for her assistance in proofreading the chapter drafts and offering meticulous review and editing feedback.

Teresa Shellenbarger, PhD, RN, CNE, ANEF

Contents

Development of the Core Competencies of Clinical Nurse Educators

Linda S. Christensen, EdD, JD, RN, CNE

Larry E. Simmons, PhD, RN, CNE, NEA-BC

As a leader in excellence in nursing education, the National League for Nursing (NLN) has consistently been at the forefront of initiatives that advance the role of nursing and nurse educators. In the early 2000s, the NLN identified the need to articulate nursing education as an advanced practice role and began a series of initiatives to recognize nursing education as a specialty. At that time, there was a need to clearly convey the knowledge, skills, and attitudes for the nurse educator role in academia. In 2004, the work began to identify the core competencies for the "full scope" of the academic nurse educator role.

The full scope of the academic nurse educator role has been published in various NLN documents, including the NLN Certification Commission's publication *The Scope of Practice for Academic Nurse Educators* (NLN, 2012) and *Nurse Educator Competencies: Creating an Evidence-based Practice for Nurse Educators* (Halstead, 2007). However, not all academic nurse educators function in the full scope of the academic nurse educator role. Some nurse educators have a scope of practice that is limited to providing clinical education experiences that typically take place in health care settings and are frequently outside the formal academic environment. As of 2015, the specific role of the clinical nurse educator had not been clearly explained, nor had competencies for this role been identified. Thus, early in 2015, the initial steps to identify core competencies of the academic clinical nurse educator began. This publication presents the results of an NLN task group that identified the role and core competencies of the academic clinical nurse educator.

The original academic nurse educator competencies were drawn from an extensive review of the literature (Halstead, 2007). Those core competencies identified the scope of practice for the academic nurse educator role and were further articulated by corresponding task statements. National practice analyses focused on the academic nurse educator role were conducted by the NLN in 2005 and 2011, and further validated the competencies originally identified from the literature. The NLN created a nurse educator certification exam following the first practice analysis.

According to B. Malone (personal communication, June 1, 2017), since the first certification exam was administered in 2005, more than 5,800 academic nurse educators have earned the credential of certified nurse educator (CNE). Yet very little research has been conducted on nurse education certification and the potential effects of certification on student outcomes (Christensen, 2015). Much of CNE research has been descriptive, such as the identification of variables associated with passing the CNE exam (Ortelli, 2012, 2016), the identification of variables associated with failing the CNE exam (Lundeen, 2014, 2018), and perceived levels of core competency attainment by CNEs (Higbie, 2010). Despite the scant research associated with the academic nurse educator competencies, their identification has had an impact on nursing education and educational practice. Many graduate nursing programs have used the competencies as a basis for the development of graduate nursing education courses, academic nurse educator position descriptions, and academic nurse educator performance evaluations. Their widespread acceptance and diverse use suggest that they help fill a critical gap in nursing education.

Various studies have indicated a shortage of academic nurse educators. A recent report from the American Association of Colleges of Nursing (2017) stated that nursing program enrollments have been restricted due to an academic nurse educator shortage. The NLN 2014–2015 Faculty Census Survey (NLN, 2016) identified vacancies in nursing programs ranging from 2 percent to 34 percent, depending on the type of nursing education program. The Faculty Census Survey also identified that 83 percent of nursing programs sought to hire new faculty, and that the leading difficulty in hiring was an insufficient number of qualified faculty (NLN, 2016). The shortage of nurse faculty was also listed as the major cause of nursing school capacity constraints by the National Advisory Council on Nurse Education and Practice (2010).

Nursing programs have sought to fill the hiring void by employing clinical educators. In the current environment of nursing education, clinical nurse educators are critically needed to work with nursing students in the clinical role. To provide a safe environment for both students and patients, clinical time needs to be an intensive learning time of application of theory to student clinical activities with professional supervision.

Up to this point in time, the role of the clinical nurse educator has been ill-defined and varies from academic institution to academic institution. The terminology associated with this role can be confusing, as educators may use titles such as *adjunct, part-time, temporary, preceptor, contingent,* or *sessional faculty.* Some academic clinical nurse educators may be employed as full-time faculty who teach in the clinical setting for part of their workload, whereas others may be employed as part-time faculty with teaching assignments limited to clinical courses. Job titles may be prescribed by institutions and state regulations governing academic nursing education programs and can lead to these varied titles. Frequently, faculty teaching in this clinical-only teaching role are clinical nurses who agree to teach a group (or groups) of students for their clinical coursework. They may be inexperienced in the faculty role and new to academic nursing. They may or may not be actively involved with the academic institution and the regular academic faculty. Regardless of job title and experience, these clinical nurse educators engage in critical educational activities with students, yet current literature does not provide a consistent definition, duties, competencies, or tasks describing the academic clinical nurse educator role.

The development and establishment of evidence-based core competencies and related task statements provide a framework of excellence in practice for the clinical nurse educator, regardless of the title and expected, institution-defined responsibilities. These competencies may direct nursing programs and guide faculty development initiatives. Consistent application of the core competencies and task statements could also provide validity for the institutional performance evaluation of faculty performing in the role of the clinical nurse educator.

The idea for an examination of the role of the academic clinical nurse educator began in a conversation regarding CNE competencies, certification, and the impact on clinical nurse educators. The idea emerged from this conversation that CNE competencies were developed with a focus on the full scope of the role of the academic nurse educator, which is not necessarily the same role that many clinical nurse educators fulfill. Three brainstorming meetings with senior nursing leaders of the NLN resulted in the creation of a task group to examine the role of the clinical nurse educator through a comprehensive literature review. A doctoral nursing student was engaged to conduct a systematic review of the literature on the role and submit that report back to the NLN. As the literature available was limited in scope, a decision was made to expand the literature review past the usual 5-year limit to 2004. Literature earlier than 2004 was not considered.

Multiple NLN personnel then identified persons who might be invited to serve on a task group to further analyze and develop the findings from the literature review into potential competencies and task statements related to the role of the clinical nurse educator. Ten potential task group members were contacted to ascertain interest in this work. The strategy for choosing the 10 potential task group members involved geographical location, types of program involvement, and experience in supervising students in clinical settings; having representatives from clinical education settings, including staff development, was also considered important. Six individuals accepted the challenge. NLN staff also became part of the task group, particularly those with intimate knowledge of the development of the original academic nurse educator competencies.

The first meeting of the task group, with the six invitees and NLN leaders, was held at the NLN offices. The articles found through the systematic literature review were shared with task group members for intensive review and the identification of concepts related to the clinical nurse educator role. To develop core competencies, a series of in-person meetings and telephone conference calls followed. This iterative process led to the identification and refinement of six competencies. Using the literature to guide the work, the group then engaged in the process of developing task statements, refining, revising, and, at times, removing statements. The result was a description of the clinical nurse educator role that contained six competencies with related task statements.

The next step in the process involved verification. The drafted core competencies with task statements were placed on the NLN website, and over 8 weeks, members of the NLN were asked to share comments. Thousands of comments were received and downloaded into a Word document. The HyperRESEARCH™ computer software program was then used to analyze the textual data. The system allows for the coding of words or phrases and the identification of recurrent themes. The themes are reviewed and compared to the codes for accuracy. The resulting themes were presented to the task group for review and further refinement, and a final document of competencies and task statements was produced.

The identification of academic clinical nurse educator competencies clearly articulates the scope of practice for this role. As done previously with the full-scope academic nurse educator competencies, the clinical nurse educator competencies may be useful to incorporate into courses that prepare graduate nurse educators. They may also be used to develop orientation materials for clinical nurse educators and guide evaluation of their performance in the clinical nurse educator role. In addition, the competencies can provide a basis for ongoing continuing education. And perhaps most significant, the identification of academic clinical nurse educator competencies provides the first and only standards of practice for this role, which will enhance the effective education of students in the academic clinical education setting and their professional nursing practice.

The development of core competencies of the clinical nurse educator will help define the professional role of faculty serving in this position. The core competencies provide a consistent framework for practice and the requirements for the provision of excellent clinical education for today's nursing students. The competencies address the relationships that clinical nurse educators need to establish and maintain with institutional staff and other faculty. These competencies can serve as a guide to the essential knowledge, skills, and attitudes needed in the clinical nurse educator role.

Describing and supporting the clinical educator role should be viewed as the framing and role modeling of excellent clinical instruction and supervision of nursing students. These students will eventually become the workforce of professional nursing in a safe and effective care environment. The outcome of excellence in education will impact excellence in nursing care for patients and society.

References

American Association of Colleges of Nursing. (2017). *Nursing shortage fact sheet.* Retrieved from http://www.aacn.nche.edu/media-relations/NrsgShortageFS.pdf

Christensen, L. (2015). *Factors related to success on the certified nurse educator (CNE®) examination* (Doctoral dissertation). Available from ProQuest Dissertations and Theses database. (UMI No. 3708579).

Halstead, J. A. (2007). *Nurse educator competencies: Creating an evidence-based practice for nurse educators.* New York, NY: National League for Nursing.

Higbie, J. (2010). *Perceived levels of nurse educators' attainment of NLN core competencies* (Doctoral dissertation). Available from ProQuest Dissertations and Theses. (UMI No. 3424511).

Lundeen, J. D. (2014). *Analysis of unsuccessful candidate performance on the certified nurse educator examination* (Doctoral dissertation). Available from ProQuest Dissertations and Theses. (UMI No. 3683685).

Lundeen, J. D. (2018). Analysis of first-time unsuccessful attempts on the certified nurse educator examination. *Nursing Education Perspectives, 39*(2), 72–79.

National Advisory Council on Nurse Education and Practice. (2010). *Addressing new challenges facing nursing education: Solutions for a transforming healthcare environment.* Retrieved from https://www.hrsa.gov/

advisorycommittees/bhpradvisory/nacnep/
Reports/eighthreport.pdf
National League for Nursing. (2012). *The scope
of practice for academic nurse educators.*
New York, NY: Author.
National League for Nursing. (2016). *Faculty
census survey 2014–2015.* Retrieved from
http://www.nln.org/newsroom/nursing-edu-
cation-statistics/annual-survey-of-schools-
of-nursing-academic-year-2015–2016

Ortelli, T. (2012). *Evaluating the knowledge of
those who teach: An analysis of candidates'
performance on the certified nurse educator
(CNE®) examination* (Doctoral dissertation).
Available from ProQuest Dissertations and
Theses database. (UMI No. 3617863).
Ortelli, T. (2016). Candidates' first-time performance on the certified nurse educator
examination. *Nursing Education Perspectives, 37*(4), 189–193.

2

Function Within the Education and Health Care Environments

Teresa Shellenbarger, PhD, RN, CNE, ANEF

Clinical nurse educators teaching in academic programs must juggle multiple demands and responsibilities. They straddle work worlds in academia and health care institutions and face pressure to meet the needs of students, patients, health care providers, educational administrators, faculty colleagues, and others. Serving as culture brokers, they act as guides and advocates for students as they learn to navigate the complex health care environment (Oermann, Shellenbarger, & Gaberson, 2018). These clinical nurse educators encounter multiple demands as they confront challenging issues in health care, such as increased patient acuity, an aging and diverse patient population with chronic and multiple health conditions, and a complex delivery system. They work with novice students to ensure that they deliver quality care in a safe manner.

Adding to the difficulties that clinical nurse educators encounter, they must also effectively interact with staff in the health care setting and develop alliances with nurses, physicians, and other allied health care providers to obtain the support they need for teaching and access to the clinical setting. Unfortunately, the health care setting faces tightening budgets, concerns over medical insurance and financial reimbursements, staffing shortages, and anticipated workforce retirements. These and other factors are causing additional pressure in health care and ultimately impact the work of the clinical nurse educator.

The clinical nurse educator must also interact within the confines of the academic setting. Many institutions of higher education face budgetary constraints and limited resources, a shrinking pool of qualified faculty, and growing enrollments of students with diverse backgrounds and needs. They also face a rapid growth of knowledge and technology in educational and health care settings. Compounding the challenges even further, clinical nurse educators must collaborate with other academic faculty and negotiate educational responsibilities such as changes to the curriculum. These conditions mean that clinical nurse educators face a host of challenges that impact their ability to function effectively within the clinical and educational environments.

Clinical nurse educators may feel the pressure to achieve outcomes such as satisfactory NCLEX-RN pass rates, ensure adequate student retention, and have students achieve selected learning outcomes. To function effectively and provide quality clinical instruction, they are challenged to bridge diverse agencies and expectations and work effectively with others. Dahlke, Baumbusch, Affleck, and Kwon (2012) suggest that the clinical nurse educator role "is complex, requiring interpersonal skills to manage students, staff nurses and patients' needs, in addition to having clinical and teaching expertise" (p. 692). Although many clinical nurse educators bring clinical practice expertise and experience to the teaching role, some lack the advanced educational preparation and background in pedagogical techniques and evaluation strategies that would help them address the complex issues in nursing academia. To further compound the problem, nursing programs may not offer adequate orientation, mentoring, support, or supervision for those in the clinical nurse educator role.

The nursing literature uses a variety of terms that describe clinical nurse educators. These terms may vary depending on the institution, hours worked, geographic setting, context, or other institutional factors. *Adjunct faculty, casual employee, part-time faculty, contingent faculty,* and *sessional teachers* are a few of the diverse terms found in the literature. To provide some consistency and make this topic easier to understand, the term *clinical nurse educator* is used throughout this book. This term does not distinguish between hours worked (full- or part-time) or appointment status within an institution (tenure or nontenure). A clinical nurse educator is a teacher who provides clinical teaching or clinical instruction to nursing students. The clinical learning environment has traditionally been hospitals or other health care settings, but for the purposes of this discussion it can also include laboratories, simulation centers/labs, community sites, or anywhere the nursing student has contact with real or simulated patients.

Clearly, the clinical nurse educator role is challenging and complex. The competencies and associated task statements offered provide direction for educators to better understand the unique role of these educators. This review synthesizes the literature related to clinical nurse educators and their functioning within the education and health care environment for the following competency: *Effective clinical nurse educators must function in the clinical nurse educator role in education and health care environments.*

The following task statements include the knowledge, skills, and attitudes (KSAs) that clinical nurse educators must develop to function within the education and health care environments. This competency includes three components: function in the clinical nurse educator role; operationalize the curriculum; and abide by legal requirements, ethical guidelines, agency policies, and guiding framework.

To function in the clinical nurse educator role, the clinical nurse educator:

▸ Bridges the gap between theory and practice by helping students apply classroom learning to the clinical setting
▸ Uses coaching, reflection, and debriefing to foster professional growth
▸ Uses current and emerging technologies to enhance clinical teaching and learning
▸ Values the contributions of others in the achievement of learner outcomes
▸ Role models nursing within the clinical learning environment
▸ Demonstrates inclusive excellence.

To effectively operationalize the curriculum, the clinical nurse educator:

➤ Assesses congruence of the clinical agency to curriculum, course goals, and learner needs when evaluating clinical sites
➤ Plans meaningful and relevant clinical learning assignments and activities
➤ Identifies learners' goals and outcomes
➤ Prepares learners for clinical experiences
➤ Orients learners to course and clinical expectations, simulation equipment, and technology-based resources
➤ Structures learner experiences and the learning environment to promote optimal learning
➤ Creates opportunities for experiential learning
➤ Identifies appropriate clinical personnel to help students develop interprofessional collaboration and teamwork skills
➤ Provides opportunities for learners to develop problem-solving and clinical reasoning skills related to course objectives
➤ Implements diverse models of clinical teaching (e.g., traditional, preceptor, simulation, dedicated education units)
➤ Applies learning theories
➤ Collaborates in curriculum development and review.

The clinical nurse educator must also abide by legal requirements, ethical guidelines, agency policies, and guiding frameworks and thus:

➤ Applies ethical and legal principles to create a safe clinical nursing learning environment
➤ Assesses learner abilities and needs prior to clinical learning experiences
➤ Demonstrates understanding of the relationship of the nursing program's mission, goals, and values to the curriculum
➤ Informs others of program and clinical agency policies, procedures, and practices
➤ Adheres to program and clinical agency policies, procedures, and practices when implementing clinical experiences
➤ Promotes learner compliance with regulations and standards of practice
➤ Demonstrates ethical behaviors
➤ Practices within legal and ethical guidelines regarding the sharing of learner and health care client information.

REVIEW OF THE LITERATURE

A review of the nursing and related literature for this competency revealed sparse evidence-based information about the clinical nurse educator role and its 26 task statements. However, four major themes emerged from the literature related to functioning in the clinical nurse educator role; operationalizing the curriculum; and abiding by legal requirements, ethical guidelines, agency policies, and guiding frameworks. The major focus of the literature involved role modeling, bridging the theory-practice gap, planning for clinical learning, and operating from an ethical and legal perspective. All studies reviewed were descriptive—either qualitative, usually involving interviews, or quantitative, usually involving surveys. Findings from these studies and the related literature are discussed in the following.

Role Modeling

One theme that emerged in the literature reviewed was related to role modeling by clinical nurse educators. Clinical nurse educators operate within the academic and the health care setting, ensuring that nursing students deliver appropriate, safe, and quality nursing care that meets patient needs. These educators are also responsible for meeting student learning needs while implementing course objectives and striving to attain program outcomes. Serving in this dual role of nurse and teacher, the clinical nurse educator has the potential to exert powerful influence on students by serving as an example of professional nursing KSAs.

Hanson and Stenvig (2008) conducted a descriptive grounded theory study and interviewed six recent baccalaureate nursing graduates to determine perceived attributes of clinical nurse educators that prepared them for practice. Their findings suggest that the clinical educator's knowledge was helpful in facilitating student learning. The graduates interviewed indicated that role modeling by clinical nurse educators was an attribute of educators that positively affected learning.

Research conducted by Heshmati-Nabavi and Vanaki (2010) studied four nursing students and five clinical educators in Iran to determine their perceptions of effective clinical educator characteristics. One finding resulting from this grounded theory study is that nurse educators effectively used personality traits in their role as clinical nurse educators. The researchers labeled this as "affection for the nursing profession" (p. 164). They described this characteristic as involving faculty members demonstrating enjoyment while caring for patients and teaching. A quote from a student in the study further illustrates the clinical nurse educator acting as a role model. The student stated that the instructor "loved nursing herself and she imparted to us the feeling that we need to see to the patients' needs" (p. 164). The instructor role models appropriate professional nursing behaviors while functioning in the clinical nurse educator role.

Clinical nurse educators' ability to link clinical competency to other knowledge is another aspect of role modeling. A study conducted in China by Hou, Zhu, and Zheng (2011) also reveals the importance of role modeling by clinical nurse educators. These researchers developed and psychometrically tested a 31-item clinical nursing faculty competence inventory. This tool was completed by 218 participants from six universities located in China. Both clinical teachers and students highly rated items such as serving as a role model, offering reliable clinical judgments, and demonstrating professional knowledge and competence as important functions for clinical educators.

Clinical nurse educators also role model effective working relationships with other members of the health care team. In the United States, Poindexter (2013) conducted

a cross-sectional survey of 374 nursing program administrators in 48 states to identify minimal proficiency of entry-level nurse educator competencies needed to teach.
Poindexter categorized items into domains that were based upon a literature review
and National League for Nursing (NLN) core competencies of academic nurse educators. Participants identified the need for clinical educators to communicate and collaborate with others in the health care setting and to role model positive professional
work relationships. This collaboration with others in the health care setting emerged as
an important aspect of the clinical nurse educator role.

Other researchers also discuss the importance of professional work relationships
in the clinical nurse educator role. Zakari, Hamadi, and Salem (2014) used case study
research to develop an understanding of clinical instructors' application of research-
based teaching and use of pedagogy. Data were obtained from a variety of methods,
including interviews with 20 clinical nurse teachers, observations, field notes, and written reflections. The authors suggest that interprofessional models of clinical teaching
might aid in understanding nurses' contribution to patient care. Partnership or collaboration with other disciplines, as well as between practice and education, is recommended. Although not described as role modeling, establishing these interprofessional
work relationships will be important for students to emulate, as they will encounter
interdisciplinary practice opportunities upon graduation.

Clinical nurse educators not only demonstrate clinical knowledge and expertise as
part of their role modeling but also role model attitudes. Hossein, Fatemeh, Fatemeh,
Katri, and Tahereh (2010) conducted a grounded theory study that explored teaching style in clinical nurse educators. One theme that emerged from interviews with 15
teachers in Iran involved role modeling by the clinical educators. Participants reported
that role modeling communication with other staff and patients was an effective way to
share professional experiences and attitudes.

Older literature further supports role-modeling behaviors of clinical nurse educators,
thus suggesting that this is an ongoing and enduring theme in the literature. Dahlke
et al. (2012) completed a structured literature review of nursing education publications
from 2000 to 2011 and conducted a thematic analysis of 15 articles on effective clinical
teaching. One of the characteristics that emerged from this literature review was role
modeling for students. The authors discussed actions such as showing respect. In the
clinical setting, nurse educators demonstrated traits such as empathy and reflective
thinking for students. This concept resurfaced in work by Klunklin et al. (2011), in which
320 nurse faculty participants from Thailand self-reported their role-modeling behaviors, including showing respect for students. Although this finding may be inherent in
the culture of the Thai sample, it does provide further support for the importance of role
modeling by nurse faculty.

There is also non-research-based literature suggesting that clinical nurse educators
serve as role models for nursing students, further substantiating this theme. Girija (2012)
offered steps that educators take toward excellence in clinical teaching. Although not
based upon published evidence, this work further elaborates on the role modeling of
clinical nurse educators. One component that Girija identified as important for effective
clinical instruction involved the demonstration of knowledge, skills, and clinical competence so that students can imitate these actions and acquire needed clinical knowledge
and skill.

Bridging the Theory-Practice Gap

Another important component of the clinical nurse educator's role that emerged from this literature review is the bridging of the theory-practice gap. Nursing has reported a disconnect between what is taught in the classroom and what occurs in the clinical setting. Novice students have limited practice knowledge and few nursing experiences to draw upon to critically analyze and evaluate clinical situations. As their clinical reasoning skills are not yet well developed, these students struggle to connect classroom learning to the practice realities that they encounter. This discrepancy between practice and theory can be challenging for nursing students and for the educators who attempt to bridge that gap. However, clinical nurse educators who use carefully considered approaches to clinical teaching can be helpful in making these connections for students.

The literature has discussed the theory-practice gap for many years, but the specific approach that clinical nurse educators can take to bridge this gap is still inadequately explored. There are some beginning suggestions of strategies and approaches that clinical nurse educators can use in their clinical teaching. Andrew, Halcomb, Jackson, Peters, and Salamonson (2010) conducted semistructured interviews with 12 faculty in Australia. Results from this study suggest that clinical nurse educators who teach using current practice examples are bridging the reality gap. They teach students "the real world of nursing" and dispel the "fantasy world" of academia. They do this by telling practice stories, reflecting upon their own clinical experiences, and giving examples derived from their clinical practice. These strategies help students link practice, apply theory, and put together knowledge so that they can tie it to their clinical experiences.

The connecting of theory and practice in this way is consistent with the work completed by Flood and Robinia (2014). Although their article was not based upon their own research, Flood and Robinia provide helpful suggestions about strategies that faculty can use to integrate classroom and clinical learning. For example, they recommend providing clinical nurse educators with classroom syllabi and course textbooks to help them better connect classroom learning to clinical assignments and experiences. Another suggestion involves the use of reflection and dialogue with students during pre- or postclinical conferencing. These reflective discussions help students think about learning and link classroom and practice knowledge. Conferencing also provides additional opportunities for clinical nurse educators to elaborate or further explain content to students, thus helping them better understand the material.

Similar strategies are provided in an older article reporting a descriptive grounded theory study that used interviews of six recent BSN graduates. Hanson and Stenvig (2008) were interested in determining perceived attributes that prepared graduates for practice. Their findings suggest that various strategies, such as pre- and postclinical conferences, are useful. Postclinical conferences provide a time for reflection, summarizing, or closing the day and offer an opportunity for clinical nurse educators to help students link theory and practice. Although supportive of this theme, the data are not richly described, the sample size is small, and participants were recruited from only two BSN programs in one state.

Another approach used by clinical nurse educators to connect theory and practice involves coaching. Roberts, Chrisman, and Flowers (2013), using naturalistic inquiry, interviewed 21 adjunct clinical faculty to determine how they described their role and needs. Participants described their clinical nurse educator role as that of a coach. They reported using coaching to guide student learning and help students apply and link what they learned in class to the clinical setting.

These teaching strategies used by the clinical nurse educator help integrate clinical learning with classroom education. They are supported by findings from the national Carnegie study conducted by Benner, Sutphen, Leonard, and Day (2010). This research involved site visits to nine diverse nursing programs, with interviews and direct observational data collection with both students and faculty. Benner et al. found that clinical nurse educators who link classroom and clinical teaching create a powerful learning experience for students, whereas those clinical learning experiences that are not connected to classroom teaching are fragmented. They recommend that clinical and classroom teaching be integrated and that clinical nurse educators use strategies such as simulation exercises, postclinical conferencing, and scaffolding of learning to link classroom and clinical learning.

Planning for Clinical Learning

The reviewed studies suggest that clinical nurse educators use a variety of teaching approaches in an attempt to relate clinical learning with classroom content. For nurse educators to connect classroom content with clinical learning, they need to adequately plan for the clinical experience and select the appropriate learning activities. The literature suggests that preparing for clinical teaching involves numerous activities that can be time intensive. Creech (2008) studied 189 nurse faculty and administrators at 25 selected midwestern institutions. Study participants completed a 21-item tool to assess Boyer's model of scholarship and determine what activities part-time faculty (including clinical nurse educators) were performing. Not surprising, clinical teaching and preparing for teaching were the highest-rated items. Developing teaching innovations and teaching a skills lab were other highly rated items. Creech's study offers quantitative ratings about the educator's activities and provides some beginning insight about planning for clinical learning and operationalizing the curriculum. Unfortunately, the study does not elaborate on teaching activities or provide specific details about clinical teaching tasks.

An aspect of clinical planning involves the preparation that faculty complete prior to their clinical teaching. Schoening (2013), in a grounded theory study of 20 midwestern baccalaureate nurse educators, reports more elaborate explanation about clinical planning. Clinical nurse educators interviewed for the study felt the need to overprepare for clinical teaching because of uncertainty about students and their background. Overpreparation was done because clinical nurse educators felt that they needed to be able to answer all student questions. The nurse educators participating in the study reported the use of faculty development activities and training to plan for the experience and ensure adequate preparation.

As clinical simulation has expanded in nursing education, clinical nurse educators are spending time planning and implementing simulation experiences. Santisteban and Egues (2014), in a comprehensive review of the literature related to adjunct nursing faculty, identify that educators are incorporating simulation and debriefing activities into their teaching role. Similarly, in another systematic review of the simulation literature,

Topping et al. (2015) identify preparation as a key element for simulation-based learning. They discuss the preparation needed to teach and ensure that students develop the knowledge, skills, and behavior competence expected in practice.

Other teaching strategies that require preparation and are reported by clinical nurse educators include preconferences and postconferences, chart reviews, observational experiences, and working with nurse preceptors. Suplee, Gardner, and Jerome-D'Emilia (2014) surveyed a convenience sample of 74 educators who attended a faculty development conference. Participants were asked to indicate how often they used various teaching strategies. They reported reliance on traditional clinical activities such as chart reviews, conferencing, and care planning assignments and little reliance on other evidence-based teaching strategies. Similar information was provided in a study by Turner and Keeler (2015). Students in this descriptive study investigating the benefits and detriments of prelab reported using prelab or preparatory experiences as part of their clinical learning. Even though data were collected from 296 prelicensure baccalaureate nursing students in California rather than from clinical nurse educators, the findings suggest that implementing these prelab activities would require planning by the clinical nurse educator.

Further supporting planning for clinical learning is the case study research conducted by Zakari et al. (2014). Their findings, based upon interviews with 20 clinical educators, observations, field notes, and written reflections suggest that clinical educators not only are planning clinical assignments but also are planning preconferences and postclinical conferences.

Clinical planning activities are also discussed in an article about legal issues in clinical nursing education by Patton and Lewallen (2015). Drawn from lawsuits involving nursing education, the authors suggest the importance of clinical orientation for students and planning for clinical evaluation. Other clinical teaching strategies that might be used to ensure safety and reduce legal liability include simulation and role-playing scenarios. As with other teaching and learning approaches, these strategies would involve preparation and planning by the clinical nurse educator.

Other researchers move beyond teaching strategy preparation and discuss the need for clinical nurse educators to understand the nursing curriculum so that they can appropriately plan for the clinical learning of their students (Dahlke et al., 2012; Davidson & Rourke, 2012; Gazza & Shellenbarger, 2010). The literature review completed by Dahlke et al. (2012) provides insight into the clinical nursing instructor's role. They report on older nursing literature suggesting that to have credibility, clinical nurse educators need to know the nursing curriculum. Davidson and Rourke (2012) surveyed 44 clinical nursing instructors about their orientation learning needs and report that curriculum orientation was critical. These teachers need nursing course descriptions "as well as items about course sequence, course outlines, course textbooks, handouts, learning resources and choosing client assignments appropriate to the student level" (Davidson & Rourke, 2012, p. 6). Gazza and Shellenbarger (2010) found that part-time clinical nurse educators were forced to "jump in" and figure out their teaching role without being given essential resources. Those interviewed for the study reported not receiving adequate information about the theory courses students were taking and being uncertain about what students were taught in the classroom. Lacking this essential information made clinical planning difficult. These studies address the perceived and often unmet need for course and curriculum information that would enable educators to adequately plan for clinical teaching.

Operating From an Ethical and Legal Perspective

Clinical nurse educators face ethical and legal challenges that may impact their work. However, they must abide by legal requirements, ethical guidelines, and other related policies that govern their actions in the health care and academic settings. They must be accountable to all agencies in which they work. As a practice profession, nurses operate within legal and ethical guidelines, adhering to standards such as standards of nursing practice, rules and regulations within the state, and the *Code of Ethics With Interpretive Statements* (American Nurses Association, 2015). The health care facilities that serve as the sites for clinical teaching also have policies and procedures guiding practice in those settings, just as academic institutions have policies governing the academic work role and student policies and guidelines that must be enforced.

The research literature related to this aspect of the clinical nurse educator role is limited; however, a theme that emerged is a focus on operating from an ethical and legal perspective. The national study of professional nursing education conducted by Benner et al. (2010) found that nurse educators help students form their professional identity as nurses; these educators focus their teaching on bioethics and ethical rules guiding nursing care. In the clinical setting, clinical nurse educators expose students to issues related to ethical comportment and focus their work on the care of patients, improving practice, and incorporating appropriate care guided by ethical principles. Although not always identified by students and faculty as ethics, this work clearly approaches care from an ethical perspective. In an earlier article, Benner et al. further support that clinical nurse educators help students focus on essential ethical comportment issues such as preserving patient dignity, providing comfort, and advocating for patients (Benner, Sutphen, Leonard-Kahn, & Day, 2008). Their study recommends that nurse educators emphasize care ethics and use clinical teaching and related learning activities that help develop an ethical approach. Activities such as journaling, reflection, or debriefing about the clinical experience help uncover issues related to ethical practice and may help connect the ethical guidelines learned in the classroom to the clinical experiences encountered by students.

Professional organizations also address ethics as part of clinical nursing education. Although not based solely on a single research study, the NLN's *Ethical Principles for Nursing Education* (NLN, 2012) draws upon expert knowledge and recommends that nurse educators foster an environment that promotes integrity. It logically follows that clinical nurse educators help promote that foundation for ethical practice while working with students in the clinical setting.

Ethical and moral issues are identified in an article by Dahlke et al. (2012). Their thematic analysis of a structured literature review of 15 nursing articles published between 2000 and 2011 reveals that clinical nurse educators must "strive to do good" and maintain the moral component of care. This involves demonstrating respect and concern for others and upholding personal and professional integrity. This is consistent with the theoretical article of Girija (2012), which suggests that clinical nurse educators need to demonstrate the ethical behaviors that should be developed by nursing students. Girija suggests role modeling ethical behaviors for nursing students and acting in an impartial, direct, and honest manner.

Although not specifically identified as an ethical or legal perspective, operating with quality and safety at the forefront of nursing care is an essential component of nursing and a critical aspect of the clinical nurse educator's work with nursing students. In 2005, the Robert Wood Johnson Foundation engaged nursing experts to improve the quality and safety of health care systems. The work of the Quality and Safety Education for Nurses (QSEN) initiative "adapted the Institute of Medicine competencies of nursing (patient-centered care, teamwork and collaboration, evidence-based practice, quality improvement, safety, and informatics)" and have become a strong directive for clinical nursing education (Cronenwett et al., 2007, p. 122). The QSEN project work, derived from national data collection, provides a framework to guide the KSAs related to quality and safety needed in nursing education. Clinical nurse educators must incorporate those KSAs into their work with students to ensure the delivery of safe care and promote the development of a competent nursing workforce.

Adherence to policies and procedures is a critical aspect of safe patient care that is expected of nursing students and the clinical nurse educator. These policies may arise from professional licensure mandates and the Nurse Practice Act (Patton & Lewallen, 2015). Policies within the academic institution may also govern student performance and evaluation (Reid, Hinderer, Jarosinski, Mister, & Seldomridge, 2013). As nursing programs vary in the evaluation and grading approaches used, faculty must be attentive to the policies and guidelines that they must follow when evaluating student work. Other specific student policies may relate to clinical attendance, orientation, and training needs of nursing students (Santisteban & Egues, 2014). In the literature, many of these policy items are discussed in relation to clinical nurse educators' orientation needs and are recommended as an essential component of education programs for new hires.

Forbes, Hickey, and White (2010), in their survey of 132 teaching faculty, suggest that clinical nurse educators may receive inconsistent information about guidelines and expectations yet desire clear directives to guide clinical teaching. Clinical nurse educators are ultimately responsible for adhering to these rules. Patton and Lewallen (2015) identify actions that clinical nurse educators should take when dealing with clinical concerns such as unsafe student actions, patient safety issues, or the demonstration of critically important skills that require accuracy, such as medication administration. Overlooking these ethical and legal issues could be a major concern for clinical nurse educators that can lead to challenging dilemmas. Unfortunately, the literature only provides beginning understanding and information about this theme and provides areas needing further study.

IDENTIFIED GAPS IN THE LITERATURE

There is limited research about the clinical nurse educator role. Even in the research studies reviewed, descriptions about the role are limited. When information is provided, it is superficial and does not offer readers specific, detailed guidelines or sufficient direction to substantially influence practice. Most articles discuss the role broadly and do not address differences in clinical specialty areas. It is unclear if differences in clinical specialty areas exist for clinical nurse educators.

The studies reviewed report data collection from different geographic areas, including China, Iran, Australia, and Thailand, as well as the United States; however, it is unclear if the clinical nurse educator role in these various countries is the same and if it is representative of clinical nurse educators in the United States. Studies conducted in the United States frequently use regional samples, convenience sampling, or select participants from a single institution. Other gaps identified involve the use of small samples and exclusive reliance on descriptive data collection.

Another concern in the research literature relates to the primary focus on acute care — that is, hospital-based clinical nursing education. None of the reviewed studies discuss the role of the clinical nurse educator in other delivery settings, such as community-based settings, which are expanding in nursing programs. As health care and nurse education shifts from health care delivery in acute care settings, it will be important to understand the role of clinical nurse educators in these other settings. The community setting may differ from the acute care setting and will impact the role and work of the clinical nurse educator. The same is true for clinical teaching situations that rely heavily on the use of clinical preceptors in the health care agency. The clinical nurse educator may assume a different role when students are primarily assigned to work with designated clinical preceptors. It is unclear how this teaching model may impact the competencies.

In addition, the research is focused primarily on entry-level prelicensure RN programs, and empirical studies on diverse educational levels were not found. Differences in clinical nurse educator roles in licensed practical/vocational education, diverse RN programs, or advanced practice programs are lacking in the reviewed research literature.

As discussed, there is limited research literature focused specifically on the ethical and legal issues facing clinical nurse educators, and few current studies found in the literature address that topic. Legal and ethical guidelines direct the practice of the clinical nurse educator, yet there is sparse information, particularly evidence-based studies, providing knowledge about these issues. It would not be appropriate to conduct experimental studies on these legal and ethical issues, but even descriptive studies are missing from the literature and would clarify these issues.

PRIORITIES FOR FUTURE RESEARCH

Based upon the review of the literature, the following research priorities have been identified and can be used to stimulate research to enhance understanding of the clinical nurse educator role competency "function within the nursing and health care environment." It is critical to move beyond descriptive studies and explore multisite, multimethod rigorous data collection with larger sample sizes and random sampling (when possible) to enhance generalizability of the findings. For qualitative studies, it would be helpful to have exemplar quotes as part of the research reporting so that readers can better understand the themes presented. In addition, more complete descriptions about methods, tools used, data analysis, and findings would provide further understanding of this research. Based upon this review, the following questions can be used to direct research related to nurse educator functioning within the education and health care environments:

> What are the essential KSAs that effective clinical nurse educators demonstrate related to functioning in the clinical nurse educator role, operationalizing the curriculum, and abiding by legal requirements, ethical guidelines, agency policies, and guiding frameworks?

> What methods are most effective for clinical nurse educators to use to help bridge the theory-practice gap for students?

> How does the use of emerging technology (e.g., simulation) by clinical nurse educators aid in bridging the theory-practice gap for students?

> How do strategies that clinical nurse educators plan, such as preclinical conferencing, reflection, debriefing, and postclinical conferencing, help promote student growth and learning?

> How do clinical nurse educators facilitate learning within an ethical and legal framework?

> How effective are orientation programs in preparing clinical nurse educators for their role?

> How do clinical nurse educator roles vary based upon the setting (e.g., acute care, community based, simulation laboratory), level of student (e.g., vocational, diploma, associate, baccalaureate, master, and doctoral level), student characteristics (e.g., race, gender, age, culture, sexual orientation, socioeconomic status, spirituality), or clinical specialty (e.g., pediatrics, obstetrics, mental health, gerontology, critical care)?

References

American Nurses Association. (2015). *Code of ethics with interpretive statements*. Silver Spring, MD: Author.

Andrew, S., Halcomb, E. J., Jackson, D., Peters, K., & Salamonson, Y. (2010). Sessional teachers in a BN program: Bridging the divide or widening the gap. *Nurse Education Today, 30*(5), 453–457. doi:10.1016/j.nedt.2009.10.004

Benner, P., Sutphen, M., Leonard-Kahn, V., & Day, L. (2008). Formation and everyday ethical comportment. *American Journal of Critical Care, 17*(5), 473–476.

Benner, P., Sutphen, M., Leonard, V., & Day, L. (2010). *Educating nurses: A call for radical transformation*. San Francisco, CA: Jossey-Bass.

Creech, C. (2008). Are we moving toward an expanded role for part-time faculty? *Nurse Educator, 33*(1), 31–34.

Cronenwett, L., Sherwood, G., Barnsteiner, J., Disch, J., Johnson, J., Mitchell, P.,

...Warren, J. (2007). Quality and safety education for nurses. *Nursing Outlook, 55*(3), 122–131. doi:10.1016/j.outlook.2007.02.006

Dahlke, S., Baumbusch, J., Affleck, F., & Kwon, J. (2012). The clinical instructor role in nursing education: A structured literature review. *Journal of Nursing Education, 51*(12), 692–696. doi:10.3928/01484834–20121022–01

Davidson, K. M., & Rourke, L. (2012). Surveying the orientation learning needs of clinical nursing instructors. *International Journal of Nursing Education Scholarship, 9*(1), 1–11. doi:10.1515/1548–923X.2314

Flood, L. S., & Robinia, K. (2014). Bridging the gap: Strategies to integrate classroom and clinical learning. *Nurse Education in Practice, 14*(4), 329–332. doi:10.1016/j.nepr.2014.02.002

Forbes, M., Hickey, M., & White, J. (2010). Adjunct faculty development: Reported needs and innovative solutions. *Journal of Professional Nursing, 26*(2), 116–124.

Gazza, E. A., & Shellenbarger, T. (2010). The lived experience of part-time baccalaureate nursing faculty. *Journal of Professional Nursing, 26*(6), 353–359. doi:10.1016/j.profnurs.2010.08.002

Girija, K. M. (2012). Effective clinical instructor: A step toward excellence in clinical teaching. *International Journal of Nursing Education, 4*(1), 25–27.

Hanson, K. J., & Stenvig, T. E. (2008). The good clinical nursing educator and the baccalaureate nursing clinical experience: Attributes and praxis. *Journal of Nursing Education, 47*(1), 38–42.

Heshmati-Nabavi, F., & Vanaki, Z. (2010). Professional approach: The key feature of effective clinical educator in Iran. *Nurse Education Today, 30*(2), 163–168. doi:10.1016/j.nedt.2009.07.010

Hossein, K. M., Fatemeh, D., Fatemeh, O. S., Katri, V., & Tahereh, B. (2010). Teaching style in clinical nursing education: A qualitative study of Iranian nursing teachers' experiences. *Nurse Education in Practice, 10*(1), 8–12. doi:10.1016/j.nepr.2009.01.016

Hou, X., Zhu, D., & Zheng, M. (2011). Clinical Nursing Faculty Competence Inventory — development and psychometric testing. *Journal of Advanced Nursing, 67*(5), 1109–1117. doi:10.1111/j.1365–10.05520.x

Klunklin, A., Sawasdisingha, P., Visekul, N., Funashima, N., Kameoka, T., Nomoto, Y., & Nakayama, T. (2011). Role model behaviors of nursing faculty members in Thailand. *Nursing and Health Sciences, 13*(1), 84–87. doi:10.1111/j.1442–2018.2011.00585.x

National League for Nursing. (2012). *Ethical principles for nursing education.* Retrieved from http://www.nln.org/docs/default-source/default-document-library/ethical-principles-for-nursing-education-final-final-010312.pdf?sfvrsn=2

Oermann, M. H., Shellenbarger, T., & Gaberson, K. B. (2018). *Clinical teaching strategies in nursing.* New York, NY: Springer.

Patton, C., & Lewallen, L. (2015). Legal issues in clinical nursing education. *Nurse Educator, 40*(3), 124–128.

Poindexter, K. (2013). Novice nurse educator entry-level competency to teach: A national study. *Journal of Nursing Education, 52*(10), 559–566.

Reid, T., Hinderer, K., Jarosinski, J., Mister, B., & Seldomridge, L. (2013). Expert clinician to clinical teacher: Developing a faculty academy and mentoring initiative. *Nurse Education in Practice, 13*(4), 288–293.

Roberts, K. K., Chrisman, S. K., & Flowers, C. (2013). The perceived needs of nurse clinicians as they move into an adjunct clinical faculty role. *Journal of Professional Nursing, 29*(5), 295–301. doi:10.1016/j.profnurs.2012.10.012

Santisteban, L., & Egues, A. L. (2014). Cultivating adjunct faculty: Strategies beyond orientation. *Nursing Forum, 49*(3), 152–158. doi:10.1111/nuf.12106

Schoening, A. M. (2013). From bedside to classroom: The nurse transition model. *Nursing Education Perspectives, 34*(3), 167–172.

Suplee, P., Gardner, M., & Jerome-D'Emilia, B. (2014). Nursing faculty preparedness for clinical teaching. *Journal of Nursing Education, 53*(30), S38–S41. doi:10.3928/01484834-20140217-03

Topping, A., Bøje, R. B., Rekola, L., Hartvigsen, T., Prescott, S., Bland, A., ...Hannula, L. (2015). Towards identifying nurse educator competencies required for simulation-based learning: A systemised rapid review and synthesis. *Nurse Education Today, 35*(11), 1108–1113. doi:10.1016/j.nedt.2015.06.003

Turner, L., & Keeler, C. (2015). Should we prelab? A student-centered look at the time-honored tradition of prelab in clinical nursing education. *Nurse Educator, 40*(2), 91–95. doi:10.1097/NNE.0000000000000095

Zakari, N. M. A., Hamadi, H. Y., & Salem, O. (2014). Developing an understanding of research-based nursing pedagogy among clinical instructors: A qualitative study. *Nurse Education Today, 34*(11), 1352–1356. doi:10.1016/j.nedt.2014.03.011

3

Facilitate Learning in the Health Care Environment

Erin Killingsworth, PhD, RN, CNE

Clinical teaching has been called the cornerstone of nursing education (Hossein, Fatemeh, Fatemeh, Katri, & Tahereh, 2010), with faculty facilitating learning and guiding the development of competent practitioners (McBrien, 2006). Clinical nurse educators help shape and foster nursing students' clinical learning. Hossein et al. (2010) describe clinical nurse educators as those who "teach and transfer experiences to the students by empowering them to carrying out tasks, fulfilling professional roles and caring to patient[s]" (p. 10), thereby facilitating learning.

The following task statements include the knowledge, skills, and attitudes (KSAs) that clinical nurse educators must develop to *facilitate learning in the health care environment.* The clinical nurse educator:

- Implements a variety of teaching strategies appropriate to learner needs, desired learner outcomes, content, and context
- Grounds teaching strategies in educational theory and evidence-based teaching practices
- Uses technology (e.g., simulation, learning management systems, electronic health records) skillfully to support the teaching-learning process and patient care
- Creates opportunities for learners to develop critical thinking and clinical reasoning skills
- Promotes the culture of safety in the health care environment
- Creates a positive and caring learning environment among learners
- Maintains collegial working relationships with learners, faculty colleagues, and clinical agency personnel to promote a positive learning environment
- Shows enthusiasm for teaching, learning, and nursing that inspires and motivates students

➤ Uses personal attributes (e.g., caring, confidence, patience, integrity, and flexibility) that facilitate learning

➤ Bridges the gap between theory and practice by connecting clinical learning opportunities to course content

➤ Fosters a safe learning environment that promotes respect and civility.

REVIEW OF THE LITERATURE

The review of the nursing and related literature for this competency focuses on the role of the clinical nurse educator facilitating learning in the health care environment. The 11 identified task statements serve as themes to organize the review. For many of the task statements, limited research studies were published and nonresearch sources were used to augment the literature review.

Implementing a Variety of Teaching Strategies Appropriate to Learner Needs, Desired Learner Outcomes, Content, and Context

The literature emphasizes that when clinical educators facilitate learning, they use a variety of teaching strategies. In an article analyzing clinical teaching strategies, McBrien (2006) advocates using varied approaches to allow nursing students the best opportunity for clinical learning. Robinson (2009) also supports using a variety of teaching strategies to accommodate different learning styles. Robinson offers several examples, such as the use of "supportive learning materials, group projects, skill demonstrations, laboratory classes, and post-clinical conferences" (p. 7).

Like Robinson (2009), Hsu (2007) also connects using a variety of teaching strategies to clinical postconferences as a means of enhancing student learning. This qualitative study, conducted in Taiwan, focused on clinical nurse educators' perceptions of postconferences. The researcher asked 10 clinical nurse educators to describe a perfect clinical conference. Participants identified participation of students, discussion led by the clinical faculty, and using a variety of teaching methods as important factors in a perfect clinical conference. Examples of teaching methods given by the study participants include role-play, psychomotor skill practice, and discussion of assessment findings.

Several authors, like Robinson (2009), offer suggestions and examples of effective clinical teaching strategies. Using a grounded theory approach and semistructured interviews, researchers in Iran explored teachers' perceptions of teaching styles in clinical teaching (Hossein et al., 2010). The three themes discovered from the interviews with 15 nurse faculty are multiplicity in teaching styles, nature of clinical teaching, and control and adaptation in the educational environment. The respondents in the study indicated that teaching styles were "modified according to situation, skill (course content) and learner level" (p. 10). The subthemes for multiplicity in teaching styles include teaching by doing, teaching by supporting, teaching by being a role model, teaching by creating learning context, and teaching by monitoring.

Other researchers have also explored the variety of teaching strategies used by clinical nurse educators. Phillips and Vinten (2010) conducted a pilot study to assess how nurse faculty perceive and describe innovative teaching strategies in clinical nursing education; 71 nurse faculty participated in the descriptive study by completing a survey. The participants were asked to rate 10 teaching strategies for innovation, describe currently used innovative teaching strategies, and identify strategies they intended to use in the future. Examples of innovative teaching strategies currently being used and those planned for use in the future include a wide range of strategies, such as student-led patient assignments, concept maps, reflective journaling, role-play, games, simulation, Socratic questioning, and critical thinking assignments.

Using a different approach, Melrose (2004) provides practical suggestions about what works in clinical teaching from the perceptions of students and clinical nurse educators. Student-perceived effective teaching strategies include identification of student barriers, accommodation of different learning styles, planning activities with the students, fostering relationships between students and clinical personnel, being knowledgeable about effective teaching characteristics, and using formative and summative evaluation. Clinical nurse educator-perceived effective teaching strategies include deliberate planning of clinical activities and promoting a spirit of inquiry. Melrose concludes that it is vital to understand both student and educator perspectives when looking at effective clinical teaching approaches. The combination of the different points of view allows for a holistic approach to discovering effective clinical teaching methods.

Although the literature offers examples and suggestions for teaching strategies, the lists of strategies provided by these authors are not identical. The variety of teaching strategies given in the nursing literature reflects the challenge of teaching students with varying backgrounds, experiences, educational barriers, and learning styles. The consistent theme found suggests that clinical nurse educators should use a variety of teaching strategies to facilitate learning in the health care environment, as this will promote learning in a diverse student population.

Grounds Teaching Strategies in Educational Theory and Evidence-Based Teaching Practices

The concept of basing teaching strategies in nursing education on education theory and evidence-based teaching practices is not new; however, it is not clear in the nursing literature how this concept relates to clinical teaching strategies. Twenty nurse educators were interviewed in a qualitative study conducted in Saudi Arabia seeking to describe how clinical nurse educators apply research-based teaching and the effect of pedagogy in the clinical experience (Zakari, Hamadi, & Salem, 2014). Three themes were discovered from participant interviews: lack of knowledge of research-based pedagogy, support for implementing new teaching strategies, and how to transition from the role of nursing student to clinical nurse educator. Although basing teaching strategies in research is ideal, there are barriers for clinical nurse educators' use of research-based strategies. One barrier is the lack of knowledge of educational theory and evidence-based teaching practices. This barrier, identified by the study participants, might explain why there is not more research on the use of educational theory and evidence-based teaching practices by clinical nurse educators if clinical nurse educators lack a general knowledge of these concepts.

Further articles were found that support the need for clinical nurse educators to be knowledgeable of educational theory and evidence-based teaching practices. Hand (2006), in an article discussing teaching and learning in the clinical environment, provides an overview of learning theories as "our perceptions of learning will affect how we teach" (p. 56). West et al. (2009) describe a clinical adjunct workshop designed to orient and prepare clinical nurse educators for clinical teaching. The workshop, based upon surveyed clinical practice and education needs of the clinical nurse transitioning to the role of clinical nurse educator, included an overview of curricula, current teaching strategies, various teaching methodologies, and additional educational resources. Both articles emphasize that clinical nurse educators must be prepared to use educational theory and current teaching practices to be effective in teaching in the clinical environment.

Using Technology Skillfully to Support the Teaching-Learning Process and Patient Care

It is generally understood that in the US health care environment, technology has become an integral part of patient care. Students and faculty use information technology (e.g., simulation, learning management systems, electronic health records) when engaged in clinical teaching and learning activities. The National League for Nursing (2015), in *A Vision for the Changing Faculty Role: Preparing Students for the Technological World of Health Care*, emphasizes that nursing curricula and teaching strategies must educate nursing students with technology and about technology to prepare them for the workforce. Although articles can be found on the use of technology (e.g., PDAs, virtual clinicals) in clinical and simulation experiences (Grady, 2011; Schlairet, 2012), the question not readily answered in the literature is this: What is the role and responsibility of the clinical nurse educator in using technology to facilitate learning in the health care environment?

Davidson and Rourke (2012) sought to determine what knowledge and skills clinical nurse educators need to be effective. Forty-four part-time Canadian clinical nurse educators completed a survey rating the knowledge and skills that they deemed as important or not important to the clinical teaching role. Five areas were found to be critical for success, including simulation technology—specifically, the role of the clinical nurse educator in simulation experiences.

Zulkosky, Husson, Kamerer, and Fetter (2014) also discuss the role and responsibilities of the clinical nurse educator in the landmark National Council of State Boards of Nursing — funded multisite study on the use of simulation in prelicensure programs. Along with their specific experience conducting the national study, the authors discuss an important concept — that is, the need for clinical nurse educators to understand the difference in their role and responsibilities when they have students in the health care environment versus when they have students in a simulation-based learning experience. The role and responsibilities of the clinical nurse educator during a simulation-based learning experience vary, depending on the structure of the simulation center of the educational institution. This would lead to a clinical nurse educator needing a general understanding of simulation-based learning experiences and the ability to adapt to how learning experiences are conducted at a particular educational institution.

In a case study looking at effective clinical nurse educators in simulation-based learning experiences, the researcher asked nursing students and simulation instructors if there were similarities or differences in the characteristics of an effective clinical nurse educator in the health care environment versus in the simulated learning environment (Parsh, 2010). The nursing students who were interviewed identified several characteristics that they viewed as similar in both environments (e.g., patience, respect, teaching ability); however, they also identified differences in the availability and interpersonal relationships of the clinical nurse educator in the two learning environments. Clinical nurse educators in the health care environment can have multiple nursing students, each with specific patient assignments. This, according to the students interviewed, leads to nursing students being on their own while the clinical nurse educator is working with an individual student. In the simulated learning environment, all students are actively engaged in a patient scenario and the clinical nurse educator works with all students.

This theme of clinical nurse educators engaging the entire group of students in the simulated learning environment continues when discussing interpersonal relationships (Parsh, 2010). One nursing student illustrated the perceived difference as a clinical nurse educator in the health care environment being a less engaged overseer and the clinical nurse educator in the simulated learning experience being an engaged coach who desires the entire team to succeed. These reported perceptions would indicate that clinical nurse educators need to be able to adapt teaching strategies and how they engage students, depending on the learning environment.

Proficiency in technology may not be explicitly stated in the literature as part of the role of the clinical nurse educator; however, it is implied. Hunt, Curtis, and Sanderson (2013), in an article outlining one institution's approach in helping to facilitate the transition of RNs to the role of clinical nurse educator, describe using a web-based portal to house educational resources for clinical nurse educators and the need for clinical nurse educators to be proficient in navigating the portal or learning management system.

Health care agencies use electronic health records for data collection, communication, and health care decision-making, necessitating that clinical educators prepare students to use this technology. One way to integrate technology into clinical education activities involves the use of an academic electronic health record (AEHR) that enables students to gain active learning opportunities and practice using the technology. Herbert and Connors (2016) studied a convenience sample of 45 nursing school administrators to understand the strategies and barriers for use of the AEHR. They found that faculty training was critical for successful integration of the AEHR and that training barriers and lack of support were the most significant barriers to use. This finding is echoed in a Korean study that used focus group interviews to assess the need to integrate academic medical records into the undergraduate clinical practicum. Interview findings support the use of electronic health records as a learning tool in clinical education but also suggest that clinical nurse educators need adequate orientation and instruction to strengthen their use (Choi, Park, & Lee, 2016). Therefore, these studies suggest that academic electronic records are being used as a teaching and learning strategy by clinical nurse educators primarily in clinical simulation experiences and in laboratory settings, but adequate training for their use in teaching and learning is needed.

Clinical nurse educators are also using other technology, such as mobile devices, to prepare nursing students for practice and provide readily accessible up-to-date information in the clinical setting. A review of the literature about mobile technology use in nursing education conducted by Raman (2015) suggests that clinical nurse educators have implemented mobile technology into clinical and laboratory settings. However, before this technology can be fully embraced as a method to facilitate learning in the clinical setting, faculty must overcome clinical agency concerns, particularly as they relate to patient privacy.

Creating Opportunities for Learners to Develop Critical Thinking and Clinical Reasoning Skills

Benner, Sutphen, Leonard, and Day (2010) define clinical reasoning as "the ability to reason about a clinical situation as it unfolds, as well as about patient and family concerns and context" (p. 46). Clinical nurse educators are uniquely situated to help provide opportunities for nursing students to develop clinical reasoning and critical thinking skills. Twibell, Ryan, and Hermiz (2005) investigated clinical nurse educators' perceptions of teaching critical thinking in the clinical setting using an ethnographic approach. The six participants in this qualitative study highlighted the central concept of critical thinking as "putting it all together" (p. 73). Strategies to facilitate critical thinking included written assignments, clinical conferences, journaling, and questioning.

Using questioning to promote critical thinking is found in several studies. Brown, Stevens, and Kermode (2012) report the qualitative part of a larger, mixed-methods study in Australia with the aim of understanding the role of the clinical nurse educator in the professional socialization of nursing students. A new graduate stated that the role of clinical nurse educators is vital, as "they put the challenging questions why is this happening, what makes this different from that, what can you tell me about this" (p. 608). Similarly, in a grounded theory study seeking to determine attributes of effective clinical nurse educators, Hanson and Stenvig (2008) asked recent BSN graduates the following question: "What is a good clinical educator to you?" All study participants referenced stimulating "critical thinking through challenge in the clinical setting" (p. 41).

In articles describing characteristics and expectations of clinical nurse educators, the concepts of fostering critical thinking and questioning are clear. Girija (2012) identifies facilitating critical thinking as a key characteristic of an effective clinical nurse educator. Mills, Hickman, and Warren (2014) discuss expectations of clinical nurse educators, which include "encouraging and fostering critical thinking skills through appropriate questioning" (p. 66). In an article offering tips to becoming a clinical faculty member, Ziehm and Fontaine (2009) advocate for clinical nurse educators to use questioning to help students identify salient points related to patient care so that they may practice thinking. McAllister, Tower, and Walker (2007) further expound on encouraging critical thinking by using the strategy of "ask and then be quiet" (p. 306). Included in the clinical nurse educator role is the expectation to actively pursue opportunities and teaching strategies that support the development of critical thinking and clinical reasoning in nursing students.

Promoting a Culture of Safety in the Health Care Environment

Safety and promoting a culture of safety are vital concerns in the health care environment. For example, the American Nurses Association (ANA, 2017) devoted 2016 to the culture of safety in the health care environment. For every month of the year, the ANA posted topics related to patient safety and the wellness of nurses. As clinical nurse educators and nursing students are participants in the health care environment during clinical experiences, it is critical for the clinical nurse educator to promote the culture of safety.

Patient safety and safe practice are identified as part of the role of the clinical nurse educator in nursing literature. Yamada and Ota (2012) conducted a three-round Delphi study of the role of the clinical nurse educator in undergraduate education in Japan. The safety and comfort of the patient cared for by the nursing student was identified as one of nine core roles of the clinical nurse educator. In their study on teacher perceptions of teaching strategies in clinical teaching in Iran, Hossein et al. (2010) indicated that teaching by supporting "promotes student learning and development, and also guarantees patients' safety" (p. 10).

In a clinical adjunct workshop designed to orient and prepare clinical nurse educators for clinical teaching, having up-to-date knowledge on practice issues, safety goals, and regulations was important for new clinical nurse educators prior to taking students into the health care environment (West et al., 2009). Girija (2012) identifies one of the characteristics of an effective clinical nurse educator as being "able to transfer knowledge and skills to students for safe practice" (p. 26). Flood and Robinia (2014) discuss how clinical nurse educators must capitalize on teaching opportunities "while providing safe, high quality patient-centered care" (p. 330). Facilitating learning in the health care environment must not compromise the culture of safety, and the clinical nurse educator plays an important part in ensuring and promoting that culture.

Creating a Positive and Caring Learning Environment Among Learners

Ziehm and Fontaine (2009) postulate that although patient safety and providing quality care are vital, "if students are paralyzed by fear, learning will not occur" (p. 80). The clinical nurse educator must create an environment of encouragement and enthusiasm to help facilitate student learning. The NLN Blue Ribbon Panel and Clinical Education Think Tank, which convened from 2006 to 2008, reviewed the literature related to clinical nursing education (Ard & Valiga, 2009). This group found that effective clinical faculty foster a supportive learning environment and that through an encouraging and supportive approach, clinical nurse educators can enhance student learning (Cusatis & Blust, 2009). Although the panel reviewed older literature, it appears that this role remains consistent. More recently, a researcher in Jordan (Hayajneh, 2011) explored senior nursing students' perceptions of critical clinical nurse educator behaviors that enhanced student learning. Participants indicated that a clinical nurse educator should "create a warm environment, one that is not threatening, and create conditions to motivate better clinical teaching" (Hayajneh, 2011, p. 27). Melrose (2004) describes this environment as creating a learning community to foster a sense of belonging with the clinical nurse educator and nursing students. This learning community should be cultivated, according to Melrose, through one-on-one nonevaluation-related conversations, individual learning contracts, shared contact information within the group, and potentially pairing students into learning dyads.

Other authors also offer suggestions in how to create this positive and caring learning environment. Girija (2012) advocates for clinical nurse educators to "encourage students to feel free to ask questions or help," "permit expression of feeling," and "permit freedom for discussion" (p. 27). In addition, Yamada and Ota (2012) identify "listen to what students say," "accept student thoughts," and "guide students so that they can keenly feel the effect of care and the value of nursing" (p. 233) as part of the core role of student instruction for the clinical nurse educator. These suggestions help foster an environment that is welcoming to students and encourages learning.

Maintaining Collegial Working Relationships to Promote a Positive Learning Environment

Incorporated into creating a positive learning environment is fostering relationships in the health care and academic areas. The focus of the role of the clinical nurse educator in relationships with nursing students, faculty, and clinical agency personnel is pervasive in the nursing literature. Researchers in multiple countries use qualitative, quantitative, and mixed-methods approaches to define and compare how clinical nurse faculty maintain collegial working relationships. In addition, there are several non–research-based articles in the nursing literature that corroborate the importance of developing and maintaining relationships to foster learning in the health care environment (Hall & Chichester, 2014; Hand, 2006; Robinson, 2009; West et al., 2009; Ziehm & Fontaine, 2009).

In a phenomenological study conducted in Australia, Dickson, Walker, and Bourgeois (2006) sought to understand the lived experience of clinical nurse educators. Two of the five themes discovered relate to developing and maintaining relationships with clinical personnel to access clinical resources and connect nursing students with clinical personnel to enhance the learning experience. In a qualitative study in Iran seeking to discern elements of being an effective clinical nurse educator (Heshmati-Nabavi & Vanaki, 2010), four nursing students and six expert clinical nurse educators participated in interviews and identified that interpersonal and professional interpersonal skills were vital to clinical education. Furthermore, the clinical nurse educator must have collegial working relationships with nursing faculty in the academic setting. In the Japanese Delphi study by Yamada and Ota (2012), this type of relationship, with an emphasis on maintaining close communication and collaboration with faculty, is identified as one of nine core clinical nurse educator roles.

Studies on the perceptions and expectations of nursing students of clinical education and the educator's role reaffirm the importance of maintaining relationships. In a qualitative study in Iran (Esmaeili, Cheraghi, Salsali, & Ghiyasvandian, 2014), researchers described the expectations of students related to clinical education; 17 nursing student participants emphasized the importance of the relationship between the instructor and students and the relationship between the instructor and unit personnel as vital to the clinical learning experience. Hanson and Stenvig's (2008) study that asked recent BSN graduates "What is a good clinical educator to you?" identified subcategories of an effective clinical nurse educator as including "knowledge of the facility" and "knowledge of the students" (p. 40).

Similar findings emerge in other international studies. Researchers in Sweden conducted a mixed-methods study to describe and compare the role of the clinical nurse educator from the perspective of nursing students from two different universities (Gustafsson, Engstrom, Ohlsson, Sundler, & Bisholt, 2015). A total of 114 nursing students participated in the quantitative portion of the study; 8 nursing students participated in the qualitative strand. The quantitative strand used the Clinical Learning Environment, Supervision and Nurse Teacher evaluation scale to compare the different types of nurse teacher (university nurse teacher and clinical nurse teacher) by roles. Mann-Whitney U-tests were used to discern differences in the ratings of the students. Students who met with clinical nurse teachers had statistically stronger agreement that "the teacher and the clinical staff worked together supporting the students' learning" ($p = .02$) (Gustafsson et al., 2015, p. 1292).

Saarikoski, Warne, Kaila, and Leino-Kilpi (2009) conducted a survey of Finnish nursing students ($n = 549$) on the role of the nurse teacher in the clinical area. The researchers used a modified version of the Clinical Learning Environment and Supervision scale and analyzed the results using descriptive statistics and ANOVA. The main reported outcome was the importance of the relationships involving the nurse teacher, nursing student, and clinical mentor. These relationships were seen to foster learning in the clinical environment.

In a comparison study of nurse educator behaviors, Tang, Chou, and Chiang (2005) asked nursing students from two different nursing schools in Taiwan ($n = 214$) to think of two clinical nurse educators from their experience who exemplified effective and ineffective clinical teaching and to complete a questionnaire comprised of 40 teaching behaviors in four categories of professional competence, interpersonal relationships, personality characteristics, and teaching ability. Descriptive statistics and paired t-tests were used to analyze the data. Statistically significant differences between effective and ineffective clinical nurse educators were found in all areas, with the largest differences found in the areas of interpersonal relationships and personality characteristics. The greatest difference in the interpersonal relationships category was with the item "treats students as people with thought and wisdom" ($t = 26.05$, $p < .01$) (Tang et al., 2005, p. 190).

Relationships truly form the foundation of clinical nursing practice and clinical nursing education throughout the global community. Clinical nurse educators as practitioners and teachers must be skilled in fostering these relationships. As Ziehm and Fontaine (2009) state, developing new relationships with fellow faculty and clinical partners will take time but are paramount in providing an exceptional clinical learning environment.

Showing Enthusiasm for Teaching, Learning, and Nursing That Inspires and Motivates Students

The enthusiasm of the clinical nurse educator for the nursing profession and nursing education can inspire and motive students, as "students can see right through a teacher who is not authentic" (Ziehm & Fontaine, 2009, p. 72). When a clinical nurse educator has the passion and associated energy for teaching, it can impact student learning (Girija, 2012). One of the recent BSN graduates who participated in Hanson and Stenvig's (2008) grounded theory study described how clinical nurse educators can encourage student learning when the clinical nurse educator is "someone who is excited about the opportunities, always looking for an opportunity for the student to go further or see something" (p. 40).

Nursing students are not the only group to identify enthusiasm as an important characteristic of an effective clinical nurse educator. In Thailand, Klunklin et al. (2011) used the Self-Evaluation Scale on Role Model Behaviors for Nursing Faculty to examine role model behaviors of nurse faculty teaching in the clinical area. Eight nursing schools were selected, and a total of 320 nursing faculty completed the questionnaire. One of the three top-rated role model behaviors was "enthusiastic and high-quality teaching activities" (p. 86). Hou, Zhu, and Zheng (2011) reported the development and subsequent testing of the Clinical Nursing Faculty Competence Inventory with four participant groups (managers, full-time teachers, clinical teachers, and students) who rated the importance of 31 inventory items. One of the 6 items rated most highly by all participant groups was someone who enjoyed clinical teaching. Heshmati-Nabavi and Vanaki's (2010) grounded theory study with Iranian nursing students and faculty members identifies affection for the nursing profession as an important characteristic of an effective clinical nurse educator. This affection for the nursing profession can be seen when the clinical nurse educator communicates enthusiasm and enjoyment of teaching and patient care to students. There is agreement from nursing students, nursing faculty, clinical nurse educators, and agency personnel that showing enthusiasm for teaching, learning, and the nursing profession helps facilitate learning in the health care environment.

Using Personal Attributes That Facilitate Learning

In addition to showing enthusiasm, other personal attributes (e.g., caring, confidence, patience, integrity, and flexibility) of the clinical nurse educator foster clinical learning. Girija (2012) describes the personality traits of approachability, honesty, and flexibility. Ziehm and Fontaine (2009), in an article offering tips to becoming a clinical faculty member, advocate for compassion, flexibility, and adaptability. Melrose (2004) specifies competence, whereas Robinson (2009) outlines traits of "genuine interest, concern, caring, respect, friendliness, honesty, and professionalism" (p. 7).

Several qualitative studies highlight personal attributes found in effective clinical nurse educators. Kelly (2007) describes two qualitative studies conducted at the same educational institution in British Columbia at two different points in time (1989 and 2003) with both diploma and baccalaureate nursing students exploring their perceptions of effective clinical nurse educators. Students from both studies discuss the value of a clinical nurse educator who is calm, patient, and honest during the clinical learning experience. Empathy is identified by the participants in Heshmati-Nabavi and Vanaki's (2010) grounded theory study as an attribute of an effective clinical educator. Similarly, Yaghoubinia, Heydari, and Roudsari (2014) used a grounded theory approach in Iran to investigate the nursing student–clinical nurse educator relationship with 10 students and 10 teachers. Participants identified developing an emotional connection as an interaction strategy further defined as "attentiveness and sensitivity of the clinical educator to students and their needs, concerns, and problems" (p. 70). Hanson and Stenvig (2008), in their qualitative study, found that it was important for the clinical nurse educator to have "a positive, professional, and supportive attitude" (p. 40), whereas a researcher in Jordan (Hayajneh, 2011), who explored senior nursing students' perceptions of critical clinical nurse educator behaviors that enhanced student learning, discovered that participants determined that a clinical nurse educator should "be easy to approach and do his or her best to make students feel comfortable" (p. 27).

One quantitative study relates to the personal traits of the clinical nurse educator. Tang et al.'s (2005) comparison study of effective and ineffective clinical nurse educator behaviors found statistically significant differences between effective and ineffective clinical nurse educators, where one of the largest differences was in personality characteristics. The greatest difference in the personality characteristics category was with the item "treats students sincerely and objectively" ($t = 26.32$, $p < .01$) (Tang et al., 2005, p. 190).

The nursing literature provides an array of personal attributes that are connected to facilitating learning in the health care environment. It is also important to note that maintaining relationships and personal attributes of clinical nurse educators are discussed in tandem in several studies (Hanson & Stenvig, 2008; Heshmati-Nabavi & Vanaki, 2010; Tang et al., 2005). The identified personal attributes can be reasoned as necessary to be able to develop and maintain relationships with students, nursing faculty, and clinical personnel.

Bridging the Gap Between Theory and Practice by Connecting Clinical Learning Opportunities to Course Content

The perceived gap between theory and practice in nursing education is well documented in the nursing literature. Furthermore, the nursing literature clearly describes the role of the clinical nurse educator in helping to bridge the gap between theory and practice by connecting clinical learning opportunities to course content (Gillespie & McFetridge, 2006; Girija, 2012; Koharchik, 2014; Koharchik & Jakub, 2014; McBrien, 2006; Mills et al., 2014; Ping, 2008).

Andrew, Halcomb, Jackson, Peters, and Salamonson (2010) conducted semistructured interviews with 12 part-time clinical nurse educators in Australia, who state that the role of the clinical nurse educator is to bridge the gap and connect theory and practice. Similarly voiced role expectations were found by Roberts, Chrisman, and Flowers (2013) and Davidson and Rourke (2012) in their qualitative studies with clinical nurse educators. One clinical nurse educator, in Brown et al.'s (2012) study on the socialization of nursing students in Australia, stated the following: "So what I think the Clinical Teacher can do that is most helpful is firstly pulling together the patient care and linking that back to academia" (p. 609).

Nursing students also identify the importance of connecting theory and practice and the role of the clinical nurse educator in making that connection. In a qualitative study in Iran (Esmaeili et al., 2014), researchers describe the expectations of students relating to clinical education information, where participants emphasize the importance of connecting practical knowledge and the real world. According to one participant, "In my opinion, nursing is a practical career, but at the same time, it is not limited to performing chores. In other words, we ought to enact every theoretical principle that we learn in our classes" (p. 463). Similarly, participants in Heshmati-Nabavi and Vanaki's (2010) grounded theory study, also conducted in Iran, explored elements of an effective clinical nurse educator. These students identified making clinical learning enjoyable as an important element, aligned with the theme of putting theory into practice. According to one participant, "I think what makes clinical training appealing and enjoyable is bringing theory closer to practice" (Heshmati-Nabavi & Vanaki, 2010, p. 165). Gustafsson et al. (2015), in a mixed-methods study in Sweden, found that students meeting with clinical nurse teachers had statistically stronger agreement with the teacher role of integrating theory and practice ($p = .01$), the teacher role of operationalizing clinical learning goals ($p < .001$), and the teacher role of reducing the theory-practice gap ($p < .001$).

The role of the clinical nurse educator in bridging the gap between theory and practice is well defined in the nursing literature from the perceptions of both nursing students and clinical nurse educators. Helping students make this connection might well be one of the fundamental bedrocks in facilitating learning in the health care environment. As one clinical nurse educator, reported by Benner et al. (2010) stated, "Correlating what the students are learning in class and trying to present similar situations... very time-intensive on my part, but I feel that it is what I should be doing to help students learn" (p. 60).

Fostering a Safe Learning Environment That Promotes Respect and Civility

In addition to promoting a culture of safety in the health care environment, it is important for the clinical nurse educator to promote respect and civility for a safe learning environment. Although the impact of incivility has been widely discussed in the health care environment and nursing education, the role of the clinical nurse educator in promoting respect and civility in the learning environment to facilitate learning has not been fully explored in the nursing literature. Only a handful of studies or articles either directly or indirectly address the topic of fostering a safe learning environment in clinical education.

In a qualitative study using naturalistic inquiry, Roberts et al. (2013) conducted semi-structured interviews with 21 adjunct clinical faculty on their role and experienced needs in fulfilling that role. The adjunct faculty identify that part of their role is to provide a safe learning environment for nursing students in the clinical setting. Under the core roles of student instruction and preparation for a clinical practicum in their Delphi study, Yamada and Ota (2012) identify three items to describe how the clinical nurse educator promotes respect and civility in the learning environment: "listen to what students say," "accept student thoughts," and "create a good atmosphere in the ward, where student training will occur" (pp. 233–234). Another approach to promoting respect and civility found in the literature is McAllister et al.'s (2007) article on using transformative approaches in clinical education, including diplomacy concepts, to build community. The authors state that diplomacy concepts help create an environment of safety that encourages dignity and honor for all individuals.

Fostering a safe learning environment that promotes respect and civility is part of facilitating learning in the health care environment, as seen in the limited nursing literature; however, further studies on this topic would broaden the evidence-based strategies for clinical nurse educators to use to meet this competency statement.

IDENTIFIED GAPS IN THE LITERATURE

The reviewed literature adds to the evidence related to the KSAs that clinical nurse educators need to facilitate learning in the health care environment. However, there are gaps in the literature. It is important to acknowledge that many of the recent research studies discussed in the literature review were conducted in countries outside the United States

(Australia, Canada, Iran, Taiwan, Hong Kong, Saudi Arabia, Japan, Jordan, Sweden, Finland, and Thailand), where the role and title of the clinical nurse educator may or may not be like that in the United States. Despite the potential for differences, similarities emerge in the literature regardless of the country of origin, thus providing supportive evidence for the competency and task statements.

Many of the research studies in the reviewed literature used qualitative methods, although a few quantitative comparison method and mixed-method studies were also found. For many of the competency statements, limited research studies were published during the review period, some were older, and nonresearch sources were used to augment the literature review. Further study is needed to fully understand the current state of clinical nursing education and the facilitation of learning by clinical nurse educators in the United States.

The following discussion highlights areas to be strengthened to enhance the science of nursing education. The reviewed literature focused on clinical learning in undergraduate education and not graduate education. Undergraduate clinical education in the United States traditionally has a clinical teaching model that includes a clinical nurse educator with a group of nursing students. Graduate clinical education typically follows a preceptor model, with one student and one preceptor. The distinctions between the clinical nurse educator and preceptor are not always clear. Both are responsible for facilitating learning in the health care environment and contributing to student evaluation. Clinical nurse educators are usually seen as employees of the educational institution, whereas preceptors are seen as employees of the clinical agency. In fact, preceptors may precept nursing students without monetary recompense from either the educational institution or the health care agency. Should the KSAs of clinical nurse educators, whether an academic employee or health care–based preceptor, be the same since both facilitate learning in the health care environment?

In looking at the state of the science on the role of the clinical nurse educator and clinical education, the primary methodology used was qualitative with an emphasis on the perceptions of the nursing students or clinical nurse faculty. This is an excellent place to start exploring the role of the clinical nurse educator; however, as the science progresses, more comparative and mixed-methods studies are needed. It is also interesting to note that most of the research found for the period from 2004 to 2017 on this topic was not conducted in the United States. With the changing nature of the health care environment in the United States, can nursing education afford to ignore scientific studies of how this impacts the clinical education of nursing students?

In discussing the reviewed literature related to the competency of facilitating learning and the 11 task statements, three areas were found with limited empirical evidence: using evidence-based teaching strategies, using technology, and creating a learning environment that promotes respect and civility. Each of these areas, although identified primarily anecdotally in the nursing literature, would benefit from further research.

PRIORITIES FOR FUTURE RESEARCH

Based upon the review of the literature, further research is needed to enhance understanding of the clinical nurse educators' facilitation of learning in the health care environment. As stated previously, more quantitative and mixed-methods approaches are needed to further the empirical knowledge on facilitating learning in the health care environment. In addition to varying the methodological approach to study this topic, using various academic and health care settings for multisite studies would enrich the science. As recommended in the 2016 to 2019 NLN Research Priorities (NLN, 2016), robust, multisite, multimethod studies would also add to the science of nursing education. The following questions reflect priorities for future research:

- What are the most effective approaches to develop identified KSAs of clinical nurse educators?
- What teaching strategies are used by clinical nurse educators to facilitate student learning in undergraduate and graduate students?
- How are educational theory and evidence-based teaching used by clinical nurse educators?
- How do clinical nurse educators incorporate technology into the teaching-learning process?
- What research methodologies and measures are most useful for evaluating the effectiveness of the clinical nurse educator?
- What clinical teaching strategies used by clinical nurse educators best develop critical thinking and clinical reasoning in nursing students?
- How is the changing environment of the health care setting impacting student learning in clinical education?
- How do clinical nurse educators promote a culture of safety and civility in the health care environment?
- What are the necessary KSAs of preceptors? How are they similar to or different from the KSAs of clinical nurse educators?
- What are the most effective teaching strategies that clinical nurse educators can use to connect clinical learning to theoretical course content?

References

American Nurses Association. (2017). *2016 culture of safety*. Retrieved from http://www.nursingworld.org/cultureofsafety

Andrew, S., Halcomb, E. J., Jackson, D., Peters, K., & Salamonson, Y. (2010). Sessional teachers in a BN program: Bridging the divide or widening the gap. *Nurse Education Today, 30*(5), 453–457. doi:10.1016/j.nedt.2009.10.004

Ard, N., & Valiga, T. M. (2009). *Clinical nursing education: Current reflections*. New York, NY: National League for Nursing.

Benner, P., Sutphen, M., Leonard, V., & Day, L. (2010). *Educating nurses: A call for radical transformation*. San Francisco, CA: Jossey-Bass.

Brown, J., Stevens, J., & Kermode, S. (2012). Supporting student nurse professionalisation: The role of the clinical teacher. *Nurse Education Today, 32*(5), 606–610. doi:10.1016/j.nedt.2011.08.007

Choi, M., Park, J. H., & Lee, H. S. (2016). Assessment of the need to integrate academic electronic medical records into the undergraduate clinical practicum: A focus group interview. *CIN: Computers, Informatics, Nursing, 34*(6), 259–265.

Cusatis, B. P., & Blust, K. (2009). Student perspectives on clinical learning. In N. Ard & T. M., Valiga (Eds.), *Clinical nursing education: Current reflections* (pp. 103–116). New York, NY: National League for Nursing.

Davidson, K. M., & Rourke, L. (2012). Surveying the orientation learning needs of clinical nursing instructors. *International Journal of Nursing Education Scholarship, 9*(1), 1–11. doi:10.1515/1548-923X.2314

Dickson, C., Walker, J., & Bourgeois, S. (2006). Facilitating undergraduate nurses clinical practicum: The lived experience of clinical facilitators. *Nurse Education Today, 26*(6), 416–422. doi:10.1016/j.nedt.2005.11.012

Esmaeili, M., Cheraghi, M. A., Salsali, M., & Ghiyasvandian, S. (2014). Nursing students' expectations regarding effective clinical education: A qualitative study. *International Journal of Nursing Practice, 20*(5), 460–467. doi:10.1111/ijn.12159

Flood, L. S., & Robinia, K. (2014). Bridging the gap: Strategies to integrate classroom and clinical learning. *Nurse Education in Practice, 14*(4), 329–332. doi:10.1016/j.nepr.2014.02.002

Gillespie, M., & McFetridge, B. (2006). Nurse education—the role of the nurse teacher. *Journal of Clinical Nursing, 15*(5), 639–644.

Girija, K. M. (2012). Effective clinical instructor: A step toward excellence in clinical teaching. *International Journal of Nursing Education, 4*(1), 25–27.

Grady, J. L. (2011). The virtual clinical practicum: An innovative telehealth model for clinical nursing education. *Nursing Education Perspectives, 32*(3), 189–194.

Gustafsson, M., Engstrom, A. K., Ohlsson, U., Sundler, A. J., & Bisholt, B. (2015). Nurse teacher models in clinical education from the perspective of student nurses—a mixed method study. *Nurse Education Today, 35*(12), 1289–1294. doi:10.1016/j.nedt.2015.03.008

Hall, N., & Chichester, M. (2014). How to succeed as an adjunct clinical nurse instructor. *Nursing for Women's Health, 18*(4), 341–344. doi:10.1111/1751-486X.12139

Hand, H. (2006). Promoting effective teaching and learning in the clinical setting. *Nursing Standard, 20*(39), 55–63.

Hanson, K. J., & Stenvig, T. E. (2008). The good clinical nursing educator and the baccalaureate nursing clinical experience: Attributes and praxis. *Journal of Nursing Education, 47*(1), 38–42.

Hayajneh, F. (2011). Role model clinical instructor as perceived by Jordanian nursing students. *Journal of Research in Nursing, 16*(1), 23–32. doi:10.1177/1744987110364326

Herbert, V. M., & Connors, H. (2016). Integrating an academic electronic health record: Challenges and success strategies. *CIN: Computers, Informatics, Nursing, 34*(8), 345–354.

Heshmati-Nabavi, F., & Vanaki, Z. (2010). Professional approach: The key feature of effective clinical educator in Iran. *Nurse Education Today, 30*(2), 163–168. doi:10.1016/j.nedt.2009.07.010

Hossein, K. M., Fatemeh, D., Fatemeh, O. S., Katri, V., & Tahereh, B. (2010). Teaching style in clinical nursing education: A qualitative study of Iranian nursing teachers' experiences. *Nurse Education in Practice, 10*(1), 8–12. doi:10.1016/j.nepr.2009.01.016

Hou, X., Zhu, D., & Zheng, M. (2011). Clinical Nursing Faculty Competence Inventory—development and psychometric testing. *Journal of Advanced Nursing, 67*(5), 1109–1117. doi:10.1111/j.1365-2648.2010.05520.x

Hsu, L. (2007). Conducting clinical postconference in clinical teaching: A qualitative study. *Journal of Clinical Nursing, 16*(8), 1525–1533. doi:10.1111/j.1365-2702.2006.01751.x

Hunt, C. W., Curtis, A. M., & Sanderson, B. K. (2013). A program to provide resources and support for clinical associates. *Journal of Continuing Education in Nursing, 44*(6), 269–273. doi:10.3928/002201224-20130402-27

Kelly, C. (2007). Student's perceptions of effective clinical teaching revisited. *Nurse Education Today, 27*(8), 885–892. doi:10.1016/j.nedt.2006.12.005

Klunklin, A., Sawasdisingha, P., Vieseskul, N., Funashima, N., Kameoka, T., Nomoto, Y., & Nakayama, T. (2011). Role model behaviors of nursing faculty members in Thailand. *Nursing and Health Sciences, 13*(1), 84–87. doi:10.1111/j.1442-2018.2011.00585.x

Koharchik, L. (2014). Delineating the role of the part-time clinical nurse instructor. *American Journal of Nursing, 114*(5), 65–67.

Koharchik, L., & Jakub, K. (2014). Starting a job as adjunct clinical instructor. *American Journal of Nursing, 114*(8), 57–60. doi:10.1097/01.NAJ.0000453049.54489.d2

McAllister, M., Tower, M., & Walker, R. (2007). Gentle interruptions: Transformative approaches to clinical teaching. *Journal of Nursing Education, 46*(7), 304–311.

McBrien, B. (2006). Clinical teaching and support for learners in the practice environment. *British Journal of Nursing, 15*(12), 672–677.

Melrose, S. (2004). What works? A personal account of clinical teaching strategies in nursing. *Education for Health, 17*(2), 236–239. doi:10.1080/1357628041000171
1067

Mills, M. E., Hickman, L. J., & Warren, J. I. (2014). Developing dual role nursing staff-clinical instructor. *Journal of Nursing Administration, 44*(2), 65–67. doi:10.1097/NNA.0000000000000025

National League for Nursing. (2015). *A vision for the changing faculty role: Preparing students for the technological world of health care.* Retrieved from https://www.nln.org/docs/default-source/about/nln-vision-series-(position-statements)/a-vision-for-the-changing-faculty-role-preparing-students-for-the-technological-world-of-health-care.pdf?sfvrsn = 0

National League for Nursing. (2016). *NLN research priorities in nursing education 2016–2019.* Retrieved from http://www.nln.org/docs/default-source/professional-development-programs/nln-research-priorities-in-nursing-education-single-pages.pdf?sfvrsn = 2

Parsh, B. (2010). Characteristics of effective simulated clinical experience instructors: Interviews with undergraduate nursing students. *Journal of Nursing Education,* 49(10), 569–572. doi:10.3928/01484834-20100730-04

Phillips, J. M., & Vinten, S. A. (2010). Why clinical nurse educators adopt innovative teaching strategies: A pilot study. *Nursing Education Perspectives, 31*(4), 226–229.

Ping, X. (2008). Roles and models of clinical supervision. *Singapore Nursing Journal, 35*(2), 26–32.

Raman, J. (2015). Mobile technology in nursing education: Where do we go from here? A review of the literature. *Nurse Education Today, 35*(5), 663–672. doi:10.1016/j.nedt.2015.01.018

Roberts, K. K., Chrisman, S. K., & Flowers, C. (2013). The perceived needs of nurse clinicians as they move into an adjunct clinical faculty role. *Journal of Professional Nursing, 29*(5), 295–301. doi:10.1016/j.profnurs.2012.10.012

Robinson, C. P. (2009). Teaching and clinical educator competency: Bringing two worlds together. *International Journal of Nursing Education Scholarship, 6*(1), 1–14.

Saarikoski, M., Warne, T., Kaila, P., & Leino-Kilpi, H. (2009). The role of the nurse teacher in clinical practice: An empirical study of Finnish student nurse experiences. *Nurse Education Today, 29*(6), 595–600. doi:10.1016/j.nedt.2009.01.005

Schlairet, M. C. (2012). PDA-assisted simulated clinical experiences in undergraduate nursing education: A pilot study. *Nursing Education Perspectives, 33*(6), 391–394.

Tang, F., Chou, S., & Chiang, H. (2005). Students' perceptions of effective and ineffective clinical instructors. *Journal of Nursing Education, 44*(4), 187–192.

Twibell, R., Ryan, M., & Hermiz, M. (2005). Faculty perceptions of critical thinking in student clinical experiences. *Journal of Nursing Education, 44*(2), 71–79.

West, M. M., Borden, C., Bermudez, M., Hanson-Zalot, M., Amorim, F., & Marmion, R. (2009). Enhancing the clinical adjunct role to benefit students. *Journal of Continuing Education in Nursing, 40*(7), 305–310. doi:10.3928/00220124-20090623-05

Yaghoubinia, F., Heydari, A., & Roudsari, R. L. (2014). Seeking a progressive relationship for learning: A theoretical scheme about the continuity of the student-educator relationship in clinical nursing education. *Japan Journal of Nursing Science, 11*(1), 65–77. doi:10.1111/jjns.12005

Yamada, S., & Ota, K. (2012). Essential roles of clinical nurse instructors in Japan: A Delphi study. *Nursing and Health Sciences, 14*(2), 229–237.

Zakari, N. M. A., Hamadi, H. Y., & Salem, O. (2014). Developing an understanding of research-based nursing pedagogy among clinical instructors: A qualitative study. *Nurse Education Today, 34*(11), 1352–1356. doi:10.1016/j.nedt.2014.03.011

Ziehm, S., & Fontaine, D. K. (2009). Clinical faculty: Tips for joining the ranks. *AACN Advanced Critical Care, 20*(1), 71–81.

Zulkosky, K. D., Husson, N., Kamerer, J., & Fetter, M. E. (2014). Role of clinical faculty during simulation in national simulation study. *Clinical Simulation in Nursing, 10*(10), 529–531. doi:10.1016/j.ecns.2014.05.002

4

Demonstrate Effective Interpersonal Communication and Collaborative Interprofessional Relationships

John D. Lundeen, EdD, RN, CNE, COI

Clinical nurse educators assist students in navigating the complex social structures of the clinical health care environment and interprofessional team. These educators must effectively use their communication skills to engage in critical conversations during stressful and sometimes challenging encounters with others in the clinical environment. Clinical nurse educators serve as a vital link as they model effective approaches to building collaborative relationships and demonstrate effective interpersonal communication.

The following task statements include the knowledge, skills, and attitudes that clinical nurse educators must develop to *demonstrate effective interpersonal communication and collaborative interprofessional relationships*. The clinical nurse educator:

➤ Fosters a shared learning community of caring and nurturing relationships

➤ Values collaboration and coordination of care

➤ Creates multiple opportunities to collaborate and cooperate with other members of the health care team

➤ Supports an environment of frequent, respectful, civil, and open communication with all members of the health care team

➤ Role models respect for all members of the health care team, professional colleagues, clients, and family members, as well as learners

➤ Uses clear and effective communication in all interactions (e.g., written, electronic, verbal, nonverbal)

➤ Listens to learner concerns, needs, or questions in a nonthreatening way

➤ Displays a calm, empathetic, and supportive demeanor in all communications

➤ Manages emotions effectively when communicating in challenging situations

> Effectively manages conflict
> Remains approachable, nonjudgmental, and readily accessible
> Recognizes limitations (those of self and learners) and provides opportunities for development
> Demonstrates effective communication in clinical learning environments with diverse colleagues, clients, cultures, health care professionals, and learners
> Communicates performance expectations to learners and agency staff.

REVIEW OF THE LITERATURE

A review of the current nursing, health care, and education literature related to interpersonal communication and interprofessional relationships in the clinical setting revealed limited evidence-based information about this competency and associated task statements. Three distinct themes emerged from the reviewed literature: interprofessional communication/relationships and social navigation, civility, and conflict/stress management. These themes form the basis of the 14 task statements related to communication and collaborative interprofessional relationships that should be exhibited by the clinical nurse educator. They serve as the organization for this review.

Interprofessional Communication/Relationships and Social Navigation

Interprofessional communication and building relationships with members of the health care delivery team are essential for effective teamwork and positive patient outcomes (Cavanaugh & Konrad, 2012; Morgan, Pullon, & McKinlay, 2015; Sargeant, Loney, & Murphy, 2008). Effective interprofessional communication among members of the health care team prevents fragmented care (Lancaster, Kolakowsky-Hayner, Kovacich, & Greer-Williams, 2015), fosters a smooth transition of patient care from one setting to another (Lattimer, 2011), decreases medication errors and health care costs (Cavanaugh & Konrad, 2012; Lancaster et al., 2015), enhances patient safety, and contributes to improved patient care. Given the critical nature and importance of these outcomes, it is imperative for clinical nurse educators to ensure that they provide an environment that enhances student development and collaboration.

Research involving health care team members provides some insight into interprofessional communication in hospitals and what clinical nurse educators face when entering clinical settings with students. Lancaster et al. (2015) found in interviews with 36 physicians, nurses, and unlicensed assistive personnel in a New York hospital that these providers operate in a hierarchical relationship and barely speak with other providers. Other researchers also discuss the need for communication, teamwork, and the sharing of information. Findings from nine focus groups with 61 primary health care team members suggest that understanding team members' roles, working together, and communicating effectively are essential to health care practice and provide the information about communication necessary for teaching students in the clinical setting (Sargeant et al., 2008). Similarly, the focus group study of Robinson, Gorman, Slimmer, and Yudkowsky (2010) of 18 experienced nurses and physicians suggests that interprofessional communication requires message verification, collaborative problem solving, supportive and encouraging interactions, demonstration of mutual respect, and an authentic understanding of the role of all providers, thus offering further insight into the communication and interprofessional relationships needed of the health care team. Although these studies do not speak directly to the clinical nurse educator role, they do provide information about communication and role relationships that is essential for students and educators to understand.

Facilitating communication and teamwork-building opportunities may be difficult for clinical nurse educators given the limited time available for students to interact with health care providers. Cuts in clinical staffing, increases in student enrollment, increased patient complexity, and comorbidities contribute to the rushed and restricted interactions between students and health care team members. Opportunities for students to develop their communication skills are further restricted when students must regularly switch clinical sites throughout a nursing program and do not have opportunities to build ongoing relationships with staff. Therefore, clinical nurse educators should encourage and plan for learning experiences where students can observe, listen to, and interact with other professionals across the health care spectrum as much as possible. They should also establish personal working relationships with nursing staff in clinical agencies to develop a trusting relationship between the nursing unit and the educational program (Fressola & Patterson, 2017). These actions are consistent with prior research suggesting that the staff-student relationship is critical for student learning and includes acceptance, acknowledgment, and encouragement of students in the clinical setting (Cusatis & Blust, 2009).

Health care practitioners can no longer practice in individual silos and assume that graduates will understand how to work effectively with other members of the team or navigate the politics and social structures of institutions after joining the workforce. Clinical nurse educators should provide opportunities for students to engage in relationship building. The research literature supports the importance of personal traits and interpersonal communication skills of clinical nurse educators and the impact they can have on students and clinical team members. Heshmati-Nabavi and Vanaki (2010), in their grounded theory study with 10 Iranian nursing students and faculty, suggest key features of effective clinical educators that relate to this clinical nurse educator competency. They found that interpersonal skills are vitally important to ensure a quality clinical experience and that professional cooperation and the formation of working relationships with health care team members are important for facilitating learning and supporting and motivating students. During semistructured interviews, the researchers discovered that interpersonal skills were considered the most important quality of the clinical nurse educator.

Similarly, in another grounded theory study in Iran, Hossein, Fatemeh, Fatemeh, Katri, and Tahereh (2010) also found that collaboration, cooperation, and partnership are essential for clinical nurse educators. In fact, their interviews with 15 teachers suggest that "collaboration between teachers and students is necessary and...cannot be separated from nursing clinical education" (p. 11). This partnership involves the transmission of professional experiences and attitudes by role modeling communication with both clinical staff and patients. Thus, it is important for students to see the collaboration and social environment in action throughout their education. The clinical nurse educator must value and demonstrate a respect for interprofessional collaboration and needs to create multiple opportunities for students to interact and collaborate with members from multiple health care disciplines. In doing so, the nursing student learns to respect the role and work of other professionals in the care of the patient (Sargeant et al., 2008) and their unique contributions to the health care system and overall health care delivery. Professionals from other health care disciplines are also afforded the opportunity to learn more about the nursing profession and the role that the nurse plays in the overall management of the patient and plan of care.

Nursing students should be exposed to a range of interprofessional learning opportunities to develop effective communication skills required in the clinical setting. Learning experiences discussed in the literature include interprofessional clinical simulations (Wagner, Liston, & Miller, 2011) and transition-of-care scenarios using closed-loop communication strategies (Robinson et al., 2010) or the Situation-Background-Assessment-Recommendation (SBAR) technique. Boykins (2014), in an article aimed at providing core nursing competencies and tools for effective communication for use in the interprofessional clinical learning environment, suggests experiences with or required courses in health care informatics to enhance interprofessional learning and communication. The author draws on the 2003 work of the Institute of Medicine (IOM), *Health Professions Education: A Bridge to Quality*, and the Technology Informatics Guiding Education Reform (TIGER) initiative to substantiate this suggestion. TIGER was designed to "improve nursing practice, education, and the delivery of patient care through the use of health information technology" (p. 43). Boykins (2014) explains the importance of mastery and the use of information and communication technologies by all health care professionals to improve interprofessional teamwork.

Formal or informal gatherings of interprofessional health care students and/or professionals that allow participants to interact with and learn more about other professions and individual roles may be helpful in developing needed interprofessional skills (Robinson et al., 2010; Sargeant et al., 2008). Clark (2014) conducted a systematic review of the literature related to the use of narrative approaches for communication by health professionals in the clinical setting. The author provides a vertical framework for the leveling of the published literature on the subject and explains that each level builds on the one below to form a foundation for understanding the narrative approach in clinical education and practice. The identified levels, from the bottom, are professional identity, provider-patient communication, and interprofessional teamwork. Data from published literature within the highest level of this framework indicate that the collaboration and contributions of different clinical professional voices in team discussions or gatherings serve to enhance overall patient care outcomes. Further, input from various practice disciplines also serves to build individual team members' own voices or identities within the broader interprofessional care team. However, for these learning experiences to be most effective, nurse educators, in both the classroom and clinical settings, must be willing to change previous notions of discipline-specific educational practices and embrace interprofessional teaching and learning principles (Cavanaugh & Konrad, 2012).

Another aspect of interpersonal communication involves the use of clear, respectful, supportive, and encouraging interactions. Using clear, explicit, and fluent expressions ranks high among the 218 Chinese managers, full-time teachers, clinical nurse educators, and students who participated in psychometric testing of the Clinical Nurse Faculty Competence Inventory (Hou, Zhu, & Zheng, 2011). Of note, students and managers, in contrast to full-time and clinical educators, ranked therapeutic constructive criticism as being important for clinical nurse educators to provide during clinical experiences. In response to this finding, the authors recommend that nurse educators place more emphasis on developing positive relationships with students so that they will not view constructive criticism as hurtful. Also ranked as one of the most important characteristics of clinical nurse educators by all groups of participants was the fostering of students' professional growth, supporting the notion of faculty providing supportive and encouraging interactions. Although not based upon a published research study, the work of Girija (2012) is consistent with that of other nurse researchers and supports the importance of communication and interpersonal skills for clinical nurse educators. All authors agree and suggest that effective clinical instructors emphasize the importance of direct, honest, objective, respectful, supportive, and open communication.

Similarly, 17 Iranian nursing students interviewed in a study by Esmaeili, Cheraghi, Salsali, and Ghiyasvandian (2013) reveal that they expect clinical nurse educators to demonstrate respectful communication and behaviors and not use discouraging statements with students. The students expect clinical nurse educators to support them by giving respectful feedback in a friendly demeanor and in a private location. Students do not want to receive corrective feedback in the presence of patients, which is seen as diminishing student credibility. Communication by clinical nurse educators can have a powerful influence on students, as was found in a study by Sercekus and Baskale (2016), who conducted focus group interviews with 35 baccalaureate nursing students in Turkey. Participants reported that feedback provided to students in the presence of patients can undermine confidence and negatively impact students and their learning. Thus, clinical nurse educators must be aware that the message alone is not the only communication consideration, as the location and timing are important as well.

Civility

Although the term *role modeling* is not used in relationship to interpersonal behaviors, clinical nurse educators are indeed modeling appropriate skills for students to use when interacting with others in the health care setting. They need to be aware of how their actions may guide student development. The need for a respectful and encouraging demeanor by clinical nurse educators is mentioned in the grounded theory study of six baccalaureate nursing students by Hanson and Stenvig (2008), suggesting that this is an enduring and universal aspect of communication. Unfortunately, disrespectful communication surfaces as another theme in the reviewed literature related to this clinical nurse educator competency.

Students are not the only ones affected by uncivil and disrespectful behaviors. Hunt and Marini (2012) surveyed 37 clinical educators of undergraduate nursing students in a mixed-methods study designed to examine the nature of civil and uncivil behaviors on the part of staff in clinical teaching environments. All respondents reported experiencing some form of incivility among clinical nursing staff, whether direct (both the target and instigator are present) or indirect (the target is not present). Although the clinical nurse educators reported that the uncivil behaviors were not directed at them but were directed toward other staff members, observing these behaviors created an uncomfortable working environment for both the educators and their students.

It is commonly accepted that uncivil or bullying behaviors interfere with teaching and learning (Clark & Springer, 2010; Marchiondo, Marchiondo, & Lasiter, 2010; Mott, 2014; Shanta & Eliason, 2014). These negative behaviors contribute to dissatisfaction in school or work performance (Hunt & Marini, 2012; Luparell, 2011; Marchiondo et al., 2010; Mott, 2014) and increase rates of unwanted psychological and physiologic effects such as eating disorders, humiliation, stress, substance abuse, and suicide (Clark, Nguyen, & Barbosa-Leiker, 2014; Hunt & Marini, 2012; Lim & Bernstein, 2014). Despite nursing's foundational principle of caring (Hunt & Marini, 2012; Marchiondo et al., 2010) and the profession's consistent rating as the most trusted profession in the United States (American Nurses Association, 2016), problems with communication and unprofessional behaviors exist and incivility occurs. Researchers have examined the effects of incivility on the patient experience and have demonstrated that incivility contributes to poor patient care and outcomes (Clark & Springer, 2010; Joint Commission, 2008).

Students are often the target of bullying or uncivil behaviors from clinical nursing staff. Numerous authors discuss incivility and clinical nursing students. Anthony and Yastik (2011) used semistructured interviews during four focus groups with 21 prelicensure nursing students to explore student experiences of incivility in the clinical setting. Thematic analysis of the interview data revealed that the students viewed nurses as exclusionary, hostile or rude, or dismissive. Although students indicated that positive experiences outweighed negative experiences, the uncivil behaviors that they experienced affected their attitudes toward nursing and undermined their self-confidence. The researchers offer an explanation that student presence on a clinical unit disrupts the normal workflow, thus leading to conditions favorable for incivility. They recommend that students, as well as professional staff, be educated on institutional codes of conduct and expected professional behaviors so that they have information that will help promote effective teamwork and reduce uncivil behaviors in the clinical environment.

Incivility in nursing education does not only surface from clinical staff but may involve other students and faculty. Marchiondo et al. (2010) also examined incivility in nursing education and studied the effects that uncivil behaviors had on nursing program satisfaction among nursing students. The researchers surveyed 152 senior baccalaureate nursing students from two public universities and discovered that approximately 88 percent of respondents had experienced at least one incident of uncivil behavior originating from a faculty member. Sixty percent of the sample reported uncivil behaviors that took place in the classroom, whereas half of the respondents reported experiencing uncivil behaviors in the clinical setting. The researchers attribute the close working relationship and expectation of student performance evaluations from faculty as one cause for uncivil behaviors in the classroom and clinical environments. They recommend that faculty be educated on effective evaluation techniques and expected professional behaviors.

Interestingly, when Anthony and Yastik (2011) asked 21 prelicensure nursing students how faculty can address the topic of incivility, students reported that their treatment in the clinical setting was associated with the clinical instructor relationship and communication with clinical staff. Thus, clinical nurse educators need to communicate respect, engage in ongoing dialogue with those in the clinical agency, and clearly and effectively communicate expectations to promote a civil learning environment.

To combat the issue of incivility in clinical nursing education and to enhance the student experience and educational outcomes, nurse educators must identify conditions or factors that make incivility likely, be willing to recognize incivility when it occurs, and work to stop the behaviors immediately. As moral agents, it is both the nurse's and clinical nurse educator's duty to provide a healthy working environment for everyone, including students (Hunt & Marini, 2012). Furthermore, clinical nurse educators must empower students by allowing open and respectful communication, encourage collegial and collaborative activities, promote autonomy when appropriate (based upon the level and past performance of the student), specify expectations, and ensure accountability of actions (Clark et al., 2014; Eller, Lev, & Feurer, 2014; Shanta & Eliason, 2014). In addition, clinical nurse educators must be willing to accept constructive criticism and evaluation data from students regarding performance as an educator and perceptions of the learning environment (Mott, 2014). As difficult as it may be to hear, students can offer insightful evaluations. It is important to recognize that aggregate student feedback can suggest trends in educator performance and clinical site conditions that may need to be addressed.

Conflict/Stress Management

The third theme that emerges from the literature on effective interpersonal communication and collaborative interprofessional relationships involves conflict and stress management. Much has been written on the topic of stress in nurses and nursing students (Brinkert, 2010; Galbraith & Brown, 2011; Gibbons, Dempster, & Moutray, 2011). In fact, it has been shown that stress in the nursing profession is a global issue. Multiple research studies and systematic reviews highlight the issue of stress in nursing (Al-Zayyat & Al-Gamal, 2014; Brinkert, 2010; Chan, So, & Fong, 2009; Galbraith & Brown, 2011; Gibbons et al., 2011; Van der Riet, Rossiter, Kirby, Dluzewska, & Harmon, 2015; White, 2013). However, identifying the exact sources of stress in students is difficult due to a lack of consistent assessment tools (Frank, 2016). There is a lack of clear evidence on the most effective strategies or interventions for reducing or managing stress in nursing students to improve academic performance (Galbraith & Brown, 2011).

To address this concern, Chan et al. (2009) conducted a study in Hong Kong with a sample of 205 baccalaureate nursing students who had completed their first year of study and at least one clinical course. The goal was to determine the extent of their stress and the types of coping strategies used in clinical experiences. Using the Perceived Stress Scale and the Coping Behavior Inventory, the researchers identified that a lack of professional knowledge and skills served as the most common stressor for the participants and that transference (an attempt to transfer attention from the stressor to other things) was the most commonly used coping strategy to overcome this stress. Additionally, students indicated that stress from workloads and assignments and stress from taking care of patients were the second and third most common stressors, respectively.

Similarly, in their descriptive, longitudinal study of 65 Jordanian baccalaureate nursing students enrolled in a psychiatric/mental health nursing (PMHN) clinical course, Al-Zayyat and Al-Gamal (2014) sought to determine the degrees of stress, stressors, and coping strategies used by nursing students before and after participation in PMHN courses. Findings from the use of the Perceived Stress Scale and Coping Behavior Inventory revealed that the most reported stressors for the participants were stress from taking care of patients, stress from teachers and nursing staff, and stress from assignments and workloads. Types of coping strategies did not differ significantly between collection periods, with problem-solving techniques used most often as a strategy to relieve stress at both data collection times. The findings from this study and the Chan et al. (2009) study underscore the importance of a thorough orientation to the course and clinical requirements, ensuring adequate preparation for patient care prior to clinical experiences (i.e., foundational courses or simulation experiences), and appropriate preparation of those nurse educators and clinical staff involved in educating students during clinical experiences.

Regardless of the cause, clinical nurse educators must understand how to identify students in distress and intervene appropriately to protect both the students and the patients in their care. Students face multiple demands in the classroom and clinical setting. They may also face personal stressors that contribute to the feelings they have and the behaviors they demonstrate. Assisting students in stress management techniques and the development of coping skills is key for clinical nurse educators to foster a healthy learning environment and build effective interprofessional teams. One such technique is mindfulness meditation. In a critical review of 13 empirical articles related to mindfulness-based meditation in practicing nurses or nursing students, Smith (2014) found that mindfulness-based stress reduction strategies led to decreased stress, decreased burnout, decreased anxiety, improved focus, self-improvement, increased empathy, and improved mood.

In a related study of 89 second-year clinical nursing students in a public college in Thailand (Ratanasiripong, Park, Ratanasiripong, & Kathalae, 2015), researchers investigated the effects of biofeedback and mindfulness meditation on stress and anxiety levels. An analysis of data from the Perceived Stress Scale and the State Anxiety Scale revealed that biofeedback helped reduce anxiety while maintaining stress levels, but the change was not significant. However, statistically significant reductions were discovered in both stress and anxiety levels from the beginning of the clinical semester to 4 weeks later with the use of mindfulness meditation.

Van der Riet et al. (2015) also found in their descriptive qualitative study of 10 first-year baccalaureate nursing and midwifery students in Australia that mindfulness had a positive effect on levels of stress following a pilot stress management and mindfulness program. Thematic analysis of the semistructured focus group interviews revealed three distinct themes: attending to self (enhanced self-care), attending to others (enhanced ability to care for others), and attending to the program (practicing mindfulness skills). In addition to stress reduction, student participants reported increased concentration and clarity of thought after using mindfulness techniques.

Since interprofessional collaboration and education is now being encouraged throughout more health science programs (Interprofessional Education Collaborative, 2016), professionals may be better trained to work together effectively. Unfortunately, this may take some time, as many current health care professionals were educated in discipline-specific silos and are not prepared to handle the dynamic nature of interprofessional teamwork in the clinical setting (Friend, Friend, Ford, & Ewell, 2016). Until all health care team members can collaborate effectively, clinical nurse educators must assist nursing students in dealing with interpersonal conflict, which is inevitable in the fast-paced, multidisciplinary health care environment.

Interpersonal conflict was examined in a study by Pines et al. (2014) to determine if a simulated experience designed to manage intimidating and disruptive behaviors of others led to increased perceptions of resiliency, psychological empowerment, and conflict management styles. A convenience sample of 60 baccalaureate nursing students enrolled in upper division courses was used in this quasi-experimental pre-post design study. Findings from the study revealed that there were no significant changes in empowerment and stress resiliency following the simulation experience. Further, aggregate student scores for conflict management were in the 50th percentile, with a preference for accommodating and avoiding management styles, although preference for a compromising management style did increase following the simulation experience. Although the authors acknowledge the small sample size as a possible explanation for the lack of clinically relevant changes in this study, they encourage nurse educators to integrate conflict resolution throughout the nursing curriculum and provide multiple opportunities for students to practice conflict management skills.

The leaders of the National League for Nursing (NLN), in a 2015 vision statement, *Interprofessional Collaboration in Education and Practice*, call for reform in nursing education and the practice environment with a call to action for clinical nurse educators, as well as nursing programs, nursing leaders, and nursing organizations (NLN, 2015). This document, which draws on the work of experts to provide background and direction for educational reform, may be particularly helpful for clinical nursing education. The NLN suggests that interprofessional collaboration is essential for preparing nurse graduates to work effectively as managers of care in interprofessional teams and that clinical nurse educators can play an important role in providing these vital clinical learning experiences. The NLN also provides a toolkit, *Guide to Effective Interprofessional Education Experiences in Nursing Education* (Speakman, Tagliareni, Sherburne, & Sicks, n.d.), to offer further help for nurse educators. This toolkit directs educational experiences that may ultimately assist in the development of effective communication, team building, and conflict resolution skills. Further work is needed to understand the issues involved.

IDENTIFIED GAPS IN THE LITERATURE

The clinical nurse educator is in a unique role to guide students in the learning environment. With direct access to interprofessional teams in the health care environment and trends in institutional policies and procedures, the clinical nurse educator serves as a leader in the social navigation of the clinical setting. Additionally, the clinical nurse educator assists students in applying practical knowledge, skills, and attitudes required of professional or advance practice nurses while effectively role modeling communication and teamwork skills for students. However, the review of the literature revealed several gaps in the research specific to that role as it relates to effective interpersonal communication and collaborative interprofessional relationships.

There were no research reports found in the reviewed literature related to this competency and the clinical nurse educator teaching graduate nursing students. Studies focus on prelicensure students and the effects of faculty communication and role modeling on the development of prelicensure undergraduate nursing students. Further research is needed to understand the unique role of the clinical nurse educator when teaching the graduate nursing student.

Another aspect missing from the available literature is the influence of select clinical nurse educator characteristics such as clinical work experience, specialty certification, teaching experience, communication style, and other variables that might impact interprofessional communication, teamwork, conflict management, stress management, and role modeling. It is unclear what role teacher characteristics may play in communication and social navigation.

Attention should also be focused on research about the clinical learning environment outside the acute care hospital setting. Only one research study was found that spoke to the role of the clinical nurse educator in community settings as related to this competency. Given the shift to community-based clinical learning, further research related to the clinical nurse educator's role in settings such as clinics, long-term care facilities, pediatric sites (including K-12 schools), hospice and home health agencies, homeless, substance abuse, or rehabilitation shelters, and occupational health centers should be conducted. Additionally, research is needed on clinical nurse educator communication during clinical skills lab and simulation activities. Future studies on this subject are warranted, especially with the increased focus on simulation use in clinical nursing education. Also of note is the lack of studies on the clinical nurse educator's role in interprofessional collaboration.

Since incivility emerged as one of the themes related to this competency, further research related to incivility in the clinical setting is warranted. Although multiple studies exist regarding the effects of incivility as it relates to nurse-nurse and nurse-physician relationships in the clinical environment and student-faculty relationships and incivility in the classroom, few studies were discovered related to student-faculty, nurse-faculty, or student-student relationships in the clinical environment. Research examining effective methods of developing and maintaining collegial and civil interprofessional relationships would enhance the body of knowledge for clinical nurse educators. Further, updated studies addressing conflict and effective stress management in the clinical setting would enhance the current body of literature. Attention should be placed on the identification of stress and its causes in the clinical nursing student, effective stress management techniques that can be employed in the clinical setting, and the effectiveness of select strategies and interventions that can be used by clinical nurse educators.

Like many of the other clinical nurse educator competencies, most of the available research was completed in countries outside the United States. The studies also used primarily descriptive data collection methods with small samples at single sites. Robust, multisite research using strong methodological approaches and random sampling techniques would help to advance understanding of this competency.

PRIORITIES FOR FUTURE RESEARCH

Based upon the review of the literature, the following research priorities have been identified and can be used to stimulate research to enhance understanding of the clinical nurse educator competency of demonstrating effective interpersonal communication and collaborative interprofessional relationships:

> What are the professional development needs of the clinical nurse educator regarding interprofessional communication and collaboration?

> What are the most effective clinical teaching approaches that facilitate the development of interpersonal communication and collaborative interprofessional relationships for undergraduate and graduate nursing students?

> What are the most effective strategies for teaching students conflict management and negotiation skills?

> How do clinical nurse educators promote effective communication and interprofessional relationship development in community-based settings?

> Which strategies are most effective in increasing interprofessional communication among students and members of the health care team in the clinical setting?

> How does clinical nurse educator presence influence the social navigation of the clinical environment and interprofessional team?

> What are the characteristics of effective interprofessional health care teams in clinical education?

> How do techniques such as mindfulness, relaxation, self-care role modeling, social support, and clinical preparation that are supported by the clinical nurse educator impact student stress in the clinical setting?

> How do self-care and stress management techniques of the clinical nurse educator affect teaching and interpersonal communication practices?

> How can simulated clinical experiences be used for students to introduce, enhance, or evaluate effective interprofessional communication skills and civility, conflict resolution, or interprofessional coordination of care across all types of clinical settings?

> What role can simulation play in the preparation of the clinical nurse educator in relation to interpersonal communication skills and collaborative interprofessional relationships?

References

Al-Zayyat, A. S., & Al-Gamal, E. (2014). Perceived stress and coping strategies among Jordanian nursing students during clinical practice in psychiatric/mental health courses. *International Journal of Mental Health Nursing, 23*(4), 326–335. doi:10.1111/inm.12054

American Nurses Association. (2016, December 19). Nurses rank #1 most trusted profession for 15th year in a row. PR Newswire. Retrieved from http://www.prnewswire.com/news-releases/nurses-rank -1-most-trusted-profession-for-15th-year-in-a-row-300381241.html

Anthony, M., & Yastik, J. (2011). Nursing students' experiences with incivility in clinical education. *Journal of Nursing Education, 50*(3), 140–144. doi:10.3928/01484834-20110131-04

Boykins, A. D. (2014). Core communication competencies in patient-centered care. *Association of Black Nursing Faculty Journal, 25*(2), 40–45.

Brinkert, R. (2010). A literature review of conflict communication causes, costs, benefits and interventions in nursing. *Journal of Nursing Management, 18*(2), 145–156. doi:10.1111/j.1365-2834.2010.01061.x

Cavanaugh, J. T., & Konrad, S. C. (2012). Fostering the development of effective person-centered healthcare communication skills: An interprofessional shared learning model. *Work, 41*(3), 293–301. doi:10.3233/WOR-2012-1292

Chan, C. K. L., So, W. K. W., & Fong, D. Y. T. (2009). Hong Kong baccalaureate nursing students' stress and their coping strategies in clinical practice. *Journal of Professional Nursing, 25*(5), 307–313. doi:10.1016/j.profnurs.2009.01.018

Clark, C. M., Nguyen, D. T., & Barbosa-Leiker, C. (2014). Student perceptions of stress, coping, relationships, and academic civility: A longitudinal study. *Nurse Educator, 39*(4), 170–174. doi:10.1097/NNE.0000000000000049

Clark, C. M., & Springer, P. J. (2010). Academic nurse leaders' role in fostering a culture of civility in nursing education. *Journal of Nursing Education, 49*(6), 319–325. doi:10.3928/01484834-20100224-01

Clark, P. G. (2014). Narrative in interprofessional education and practice: Implications for professional identity, provider-patient communication and teamwork. *Journal of Interprofessional Care, 28*(1), 34–39. doi:10.3109/13561820.2013.853652

Cusatis, B. P., & Blust, K. (2009). Student perspectives on clinical learning. In N. Ard & T. M. Valiga (Eds.), *Clinical nursing education: Current reflections* (pp. 103–116). New York, NY: National League for Nursing.

Eller, L. S., Lev, E. L., & Feurer, A. (2014). Key components of an effective mentoring relationship: A qualitative study. *Nurse Education Today, 34*(5), 815–820. doi:10/1016/j.nedt.2013.07.020

Esmaeili, M., Cheraghi, M. A., Salsali, M., & Ghiyasvandian, S. (2013). Nursing students' expectations regarding effective clinical education: A qualitative study. *International Journal of Nursing Practice, 20*(5), 460–467. doi:10.1111/ijn.12159

Frank, B. (2016). Facilitating learning for students with disabilities. In D. M. Billings & J. A. Halstead (Eds.), *Teaching in nursing: A guide for faculty* (5th ed., pp. 55–72). St. Louis, MO: Elsevier.

Fressola, M. C., & Patterson, G. E. (Eds.). (2017). Contextual factors influencing the clinical experience. In *Transition from clinician to educator: A practical approach* (pp. 115–132). Burlington, MA: Jones & Bartlett Learning.

Friend, M. L., Friend, R. D., Ford, C., & Ewell, P. J. (2016). Critical care interprofessional education: Exploring conflict and power—lessons learned. *Journal of Nursing Education, 55*(12), 693–700. doi:10.3928/01484834-20161114-06

Galbraith, N. D., & Brown, K. E. (2011). Assessing intervention effectiveness for reducing stress in student nurses: Quantitative systematic review. *Journal of Advanced Nursing, 67*(4), 709–721. doi:10.1111/j.1365-2648.2010.05549.x

Gibbons, C., Dempster, M., & Moutray, M (2011). Stress, coping and satisfaction in nursing students. *Journal of Advanced Nursing, 67*(3), 621–632. doi:10.1011/j.1365-2648/2010.05495x

Girija, K. M. (2012). Effective clinical instructor: A step toward excellence in clinical teaching. *International Journal of Nursing Education, 4*(1), 25–27.

Hanson, K. J., & Stenvig, T. E. (2008). The good clinical nursing educator and the baccalaureate nursing clinical experience: Attributes and praxis. *Journal of Nursing Education, 47*(1), 38–42.

Heshmati-Nabavi, F., & Vanaki, Z. (2010). Professional approach: The key feature of effective clinical educator in Iran. *Nurse Education Today, 30*(2), 163–168. doi:10.1016/j.nedt.2009.07.010

Hossein, K. M., Fatemeh, D., Fatemeh, O. S., Katri, V., & Tahereh, B. (2010). Teaching style in clinical nursing education: A qualitative study of Iranian nursing teachers' experiences. *Nurse Education in Practice, 10*(1), 8–12. doi:10.1016/j.nepr.2009.01.016

Hou, X., Zhu, D., & Zheng, M. (2011). Clinical Nursing Faculty Competence

Inventory—development and psychometric testing. *Journal of Advanced Nursing, 67*(5), 1109–1117. doi:10.1111/j.1365-2648.2010.05520.x

Hunt, C., & Marini, Z. A. (2012). Incivility in the practice environment: A perspective from clinical nursing teachers. *Nurse Education in Practice, 12*(6), 366–370. doi:10.1016/j.nepr.2012.05.001

Interprofessional Education Collaborative. (2016, July 11). *Interprofessional Education Collaborative releases revised set of core competencies* [News release]. Retrieved from https://www.ipecollaborative.org/news-releases.html

Joint Commission. (2008). *Sentinel Event Alert, Issue 40: Behaviors that undermine a culture of safety*. Retrieved from https://www.jointcommission.org/sentinel_event_alert_is-sue_40_behaviors_that_undermine_a_cul-ture_of_safety/

Lancaster, G., Kolakowsky-Hayner, S., Kovac-ich, J., & Greer-Williams, N. (2015). Interdis-ciplinary communication and collaboration among physicians, nurses, and unlicensed assistive personnel. *Journal of Nursing Schol-arship, 47*(3), 275–284. doi:10.1111/jnu.12130

Lattimer, C. (2011). When it comes to transitions in patient care, effective com-munication can make all the difference. *Generations, 35*(1), 69–72.

Lim, F. A., & Bernstein, I. (2014). Civility and workplace bullying: Resonance of Nightin-gale's persona and current best practices. *Nursing Forum, 49*(2), 124–129.

Luparell, S. (2011). Incivility in nursing: The connection between academia and clinical settings. *Critical Care Nurse, 31*(2), 92–95. doi:10.4037/ccn2011171

Marchiondo, K., Marchiondo, L. A., & Lasiter, S. (2010). Faculty incivility: Effects on pro-gram satisfaction of BSN students. *Journal of Nursing Education, 49*(11), 608–614. doi:10.3928/01484834-20100524-05

Morgan, S., Pullon, S., & McKinlay, E. (2015). Observation of interprofessional collabora-tive practice in primary care teams: An inte-grative literature review. *International Journal of Nursing Studies, 52*(7), 1217–1230. doi:10.1016/j.ijnurstu.2015.03.008

Mott, J. (2014). Undergraduate nursing student experiences with faculty bullies. *Nurse Educator, 39*(3), 143–148. doi:10.1097/NNE.0000000000000038

National League for Nursing. (2015). *Interpro-fessional collaboration in education and practice*. Retrieved from http://www.nln.org/newsroom/nln-position-documents/nln-living-documents

Pines, E. W., Rauschhuber, M. L., Cook, J. D., Norgan, G. H., Canchola, L., Richardson, C., & Jones, M. (2014). Enhancing resilience, empowerment, and conflict management among baccalaureate students: Outcomes of a pilot study. *Nurse Educator, 39*(2), 85–90. doi:10.1097/NNE.0000000000000023

Ratanasiripong, P., Park, J. F., Ratanasiripong, N., & Kathalae, D. (2015). Stress and anxiety management in nursing students: Biofeed-back and mindfulness meditation. *Journal of Nursing Education, 54*(9), 520–524. doi:10.3928/01484834-20150814-07

Robinson, F. P., Gorman, G., Slimmer, L. W., & Yudkowsky, R. (2010). Perceptions of effective and ineffective nurse-physician communication in hospitals. *Nursing Forum, 45*(3), 206–216.

Sargeant, J., Loney, E., & Murphy, G. (2008). Effective interprofessional teams: "Contact is not enough" to build a team. *Journal of Continuing Education in the Health Professions, 28*(4), 228–234. doi:10.1002/chp.189

Sercekus, P., & Baskale, H. (2016). Nursing students' perceptions about clinical learning environment in Turkey. *Nurse Education in Practice, 17*(2016), 134–138. doi:10.1016/j.nepr.2015.12.008

Shanta, L. L., & Eliason, A. R. M. (2014). Application of an empowerment model to improve civility in nursing education. *Nurse Education in Practice, 14*(1), 82–86. doi:10.1016/j.nepr.2013.06.009

Smith, S. A. (2014). Mindfulness-based stress reduction: An intervention to enhance the effectiveness of nurses' coping with work-related stress. *International Journal of Nursing Knowledge, 25*(2), 119–130.

Speakman, E., Tagliareni, E., Sherburne, A., & Sicks, S. (n.d.). *Guide to effective interprofessional education experiences in nursing education* [Toolkit]. Retrieved from http://www.nln.org/docs/default-source/default-document-library/ipe-toolkit-krk-012716.pdf?sfvrsn=6

Van der Riet, P., Rossiter, R., Kirby, D., Dluzewska, T., & Harmon, C. (2015). Piloting a stress management and mindfulness program for undergraduate nursing students: Student feedback and lessons learned. *Nurse Education Today, 35*(1), 44–49. doi:10.1016/j.nedt.2014.05.003

Wagner, J., Liston, B., & Miller, J. (2011). Developing interprofessional communication skills. *Teaching and Learning in Nursing, 6*(3), 97–101. doi:10.1016/j.teln.2010.12.003

White, L. (2013). Mindfulness in nursing: An evolutionary concept analysis. *Journal of Advanced Nursing, 70*(2), 282–294. doi:10.1111/jan.12182

5

Apply Clinical Expertise in the Health Care Environment

Melora D. Ferren, MSN, RN-BC

Nursing practice and the health care environment are complex and continually changing; therefore, the clinical nurse educator must possess strong foundational clinical knowledge and skills to be an effective educator. The clinical nurse educator brings current, up-to-date knowledge of clinical practice and skill competency to the clinical learning environment. As an expert, the clinical nurse educator translates theory into clinical practice by applying experiential knowledge, clinical reasoning, and the ability to solve practice problems based upon information and evidence.

Since nursing is a practice profession, a critical attribute of an effective clinical nurse educator is clinical expertise (Duffy, Stuart, & Smith, 2008; Hewitt & Lewallen, 2010). As the nursing faculty shortage continues and nursing programs face an insufficient supply of educators, many nursing programs are recruiting and selecting expert clinicians who have experience and practice knowledge to meet faculty demands. As Girija (2012) explains, clinical nurses serving as academic educators bring a wealth of clinical knowledge and considerable clinical skills; however, the role encompasses much more than simply clinical proficiency. The clinical nurse educator role also requires the ability to facilitate critical thinking in clinical practice and to bridge theoretical knowledge with clinical practice. Hou, Zhu, and Zheng (2011) summarize the characteristics of an exceptional clinical nurse educator as possessing proficiency and confidence in professional knowledge, making reliable judgments and decisions based upon clinical assessment data, demonstrating clinical practice ability, role modeling professional behaviors, and exhibiting clinical skill proficiency. Thus, the clinical educator must be capable of providing "real-life experiences and opportunities for transfer of knowledge to practical situations" (Gaberson, Oermann, & Shellenbarger, 2015, p. 9).

The following task statements relate to the clinical expertise and knowledge, skills, and attitudes that clinical nurse educators must exhibit to function within the academic and health care practice environments. The competency, *apply clinical expertise in the health care environment,* includes the following eight task statements. The clinical nurse educator:

- Maintains current professional competence relevant to the specialty area, practice setting, and clinical learning environment
- Translates theory into clinical practice by applying experiential knowledge and clinical reasoning, and using a client-centered approach to clinical instruction
- Solves client-related problems based upon evidence
- Demonstrates effective leadership within the clinical learning environment
- Demonstrates clinical competency based upon sound clinical reasoning
- Expands knowledge and skills by integrating best practices and standards of care in the clinical learning environment
- Balances safe client care and student learning needs in a culture of safety
- Demonstrates competence with a range of technologies available in the clinical learning environment.

REVIEW OF THE LITERATURE

Surprisingly, a review of the literature related to the clinical nurse educator competency of applying clinical expertise in the health care environment lacks strong evidence and is superficial in the description of clinical expertise. Application of clinical expertise to the clinical nurse educator role is frequently mentioned in the literature as important but lacks specifics and further explanation. A standard definition was not found. The literature reviewed specific to clinical expertise revealed two predominant themes: the clinical nurse educator possesses clinical expertise, and the clinical nurse educator should have a structured transition period for role actualization. Although these themes are mentioned frequently in the literature, they are described superficially. Anecdotal and theoretical references are therefore presented for the individual task statements.

Clinical Practice Expert

The first theme identified involves possessing clinical expertise. It has three subthemes: maintains current clinical knowledge, practice experience, and skills that facilitate the translation of theory into practice.

Possessing current knowledge and contemporary clinical experience in nursing emerges prominently in the literature as a key characteristic of an effective clinical nurse educator (Andrew, Halcomb, Jackson, Peters, & Salamonson, 2010; Cangelosi, Crocker, & Sorrell, 2009; Dahlke, Baumbusch, Affleck, & Kwon, 2012; Davidson & Rourke, 2012; Flood & Robinia, 2014; Gazza & Shellenbarger, 2010; Girija, 2012; Hall & Chichester, 2014; Heshmati-Nabavi & Vanaki, 2010; Hou et al., 2011; Hunt, Curtis, & Sanderson, 2013; Robinson, 2009; Santisteban & Egues, 2014; Volk, Homan, Tepner, Chichester, & Scales, 2013; West, Borden, Bermudez, Hanson-Zalot, Amorim, & Marmion, 2009; Wiens, Babenko-Mould, & Iwasiw, 2014). Heshmati-Nabavi and Vanaki (2010) interviewed 10 Iranian nursing students and clinical educators to understand key features of effective clinical educators. They explain that an effective clinical nurse educator has a minimum of a few years of experience as a direct care clinical nurse and is proficient in recognizing client needs. Acquiring clinical expertise is intentional and does not necessarily come with years of experience. Clinical nurse educators who are familiar with the flow and management of the clinical learning environment (nursing department) facilitate a positive learning experience for nursing students. These educators have gained sufficient knowledge and experience in the clinical setting and, more importantly, utilize this experience to facilitate student learning. Heshmati-Nabavi and Vanaki (2010) further discuss categories of findings that emerged from their semistructured interviews. They describe one category—metacognition—as possessing knowledge of the clinical environment and state that clinical nurse educators understand how care is managed and are familiar with issues that may impact nursing care and daily operations. Possessing operational knowledge of the clinical environment is a foundational aspect of teaching in the clinical setting and promotes student learning.

Possessing contemporary clinical expertise enhances the credibility of the clinical nurse educator. Girija (2012), citing previously unpublished research, sought feedback from nursing students and found that professional competence, which includes both knowledge and clinical skills, is an important characteristic of the best clinical nurse educators. Similarly, Hou et al. (2011) found that 237 nurse faculty members, students, and administrators in China agreed that proficiency in theoretical knowledge and clinical skills are top-rated items when assessing the importance of clinical nurse educator competence.

In Australia, Andrew et al. (2010) interviewed 12 sessional teachers about the perceived contributions of the clinical nurse educator role to an undergraduate bachelor of nursing program. The interviews revealed that current clinical knowledge brings greater value to the learning experience. Clinical currency and knowledge "enabled [educators] to use 'practical examples' derived from their practice in their teaching" (p. 454). Andrew et al. (2010) discuss that bringing stories from the real world into teaching enhances the environment and learning. Expressions of real-life experience are cited in earlier research conducted by Hanson and Stenvig (2008). In their work, six baccalaureate graduates from the United States talk about the importance of clinical nurse educators having current practice experience that can be used to help make assignments and offer real-life experiences. This research is older but suggests the enduring nature of the theme.

Another research study from the United States provides further validation about the importance of possessing clinical expertise. Roberts, Chrisman, and Flowers (2013) suggest that clinical nurse educators help students learn by bringing current clinical knowledge and skills to the education environment. Although not substantiated with research, some experts indicate that knowledge of clinical unit routines may help educators be more proficient in unit operations, which may translate into increased teaching effectiveness (Hewitt & Lewallen, 2010). Possessing clinical competence is not only important for student learning and faculty engagement but also highly valued by nursing program administrators. As indicated by the research of Poindexter (2013) with a sample of 374 nursing program administrators from 48 states, clinical competence is an expectation for entry-level clinical teaching positions. To summarize, it is imperative for clinical nurse educators "to be experts in their clinical specialty, maintain their clinical skills, be able to explain and demonstrate nursing care in a real situation, and guide students in developing clinical competencies" (Gaberson et al., 2015, p. 106).

Clinical nurse educators draw upon clinical expertise to provide a safe learning environment for students. Advanced clinical knowledge also helps clinical nurse educators foster relationships with clinical nurses and other health care professionals, thus enhancing the clinical learning environment. Dahlke et al. (2012), in a literature review exploring the clinical nurse educator role, found that for clinical nurse educators to find learning opportunities to support student learning, it is imperative to develop relationships with individuals in the clinical setting and draw upon previous personal and clinical experiences. Nursing students and clinical nurse educators are considered guests in clinical agencies. Courteous guests respectfully negotiate with others and keep staff and administration informed of expectations and rules (Gaberson et al., 2015).

An important component of possessing clinical expertise is the application of theoretical knowledge gained in a classroom to the clinical setting. In other words, clinical nurse educators help students transfer classroom knowledge into clinical actions and client care. Numerous articles explain how effective clinical nurse educators "connect the practical world with theory" (Roberts et al., 2013, p. 297) or bridge the gap between theory and practice (Esmaeili, Cheraghi, Salsali, & Ghiyasvandian, 2014; Flood & Robinia, 2014; Heshmati-Nabavi & Vanaki, 2010).

The clinical nurse educator translates theory into clinical practice by applying experiential knowledge and clinical reasoning, and demonstrating a client-centered approach to clinical instruction. The clinical nurse educator is responsible for ensuring that students apply what is learned in the classroom setting to the clinical learning environment, thus bridging the gap between theory and practice. Andrew et al. (2010) found that clinical nurse educators view one of their primary roles as bridging the gap between theory and practice for students and bringing the clinical setting and academia together. The researchers interviewed clinical nurse educators or sessional teachers and found that educators believed that their primary role was to prepare students for the reality of clinical practice and bring the "real" world of nursing to the classroom. A concern that emerged from the study was that clinical nurse educators may widen the knowledge/practice gap instead of bridging it by convincing students that experiential knowledge is more important than theoretical knowledge. The clinical nurse educator should take time to understand how theory informs both clinical practice and research in order to teach students how theory is foundational in evidence based practice development (Andrew et al., 2010).

In the book *Clinical Instruction and Evaluation*, O'Connor (2015) suggests that integrating theory into practice primarily occurs during teacher and student interactions with client care activities. The teaching approach used, which can be drawn from the classroom, can facilitate the connection of content. Content can be linked using structured learning activities such as problem-based learning, clinical seminars, nursing rounds, case studies, and other written assignments. Flood and Robinia (2014) also recommend using strategies such as narratives, reflection, gaming, and simulation to help connect classroom learning with clinical practice experiences. It is logical to conclude from the literature about clinical practice expertise from multiple perspectives that bridging the theory and practice gap is a cornerstone of nursing education and should be embedded in the practice discipline of nursing.

Clinical Nurse Educator Role Transition

Role transition to both the academic culture of higher education and the clinical nurse educator role in the health care practice environment is the second theme related to the competency of applying clinical expertise in the health care environment (Dahlke et al., 2012; Hall & Chichester, 2014; Hewitt & Lewallen, 2010; Kring, Ramseur, & Parnell, 2013; Roberts et al., 2013; Robinson, 2009). To effectively connect theory to practice, the clinical nurse educator needs to be familiar with both the academic and practice environments, and navigate both settings. Clinical nurse educators who are clinical experts maintain competency in the clinical setting and must learn the role of the clinical nurse educator in the practice environment. A new clinical nurse educator must also develop different skills and competencies to function as an educator. Novice clinical nurse educators must "learn the mores, customs, and values of academic institutions" (Janzen, 2010, p. 520) as they acclimate to the norms, values, and expectations of the practice environment. Janzen describes this as a transformation, or a series of movements back and forth between the roles and cultures.

After reviewing reflective narratives from 45 clinicians who were preparing for new faculty roles, Cangelosi et al. (2009) note that clinical expertise does not make one proficient in teaching clinical skills to others. They suggest that teaching "is not a natural byproduct of clinical expertise, but requires a skill set of its own" (Cangelosi et al., 2009, p. 371). Davidson and Rourke (2012) explain that without formal education on teaching and learning, clinical nurse educators will teach as they were taught, which may not be the most effective approach.

The passage of time, as well as an individualized transition plan, will assist the novice clinical nurse educator in developing the skill set required to be an effective nurse educator (Janzen, 2010; Peters & Boylston, 2006). Hunt et al. (2013), Peters and Boylston (2006), and Robinson (2009) explain how mentoring relationships are important for clinical nurse educator growth and development, and help ease the transition from clinical expert to clinical nurse educator. West et al. (2009) state that master-prepared nurse practitioners and clinical nurse specialists have the potential to become exceptional clinical nurse educators with support and education about the teaching role.

Findings from the literature stress the importance of a formal orientation including an introduction to the academic institution and the clinical learning environment (Davidson & Rourke, 2012; Hewitt & Lewallen, 2010; Koharchik & Jakub, 2014; Reid, Hinderer, Jarosinski, Mister, & Seldomridge, 2013; Roberts et al., 2013; Santisteban & Egues, 2014). Peters and Boylston (2006) and Davidson and Rourke (2012) state that clinical expertise and orientation are vital to success in the clinical educator role.

Before beginning a clinical teaching assignment, clinical nurse educators should participate in orientation to the practice setting so that they can appropriately apply policies, protocols, and procedures to the clinical learning environment and facilitation of student learning. Orientation to the practice organization/setting is vital even if the clinical nurse educator is employed by the organization, as clinical nurse educators function in a different role than health care employees. While teaching students in the clinical setting, the clinical nurse educator must adhere to policies governing student expectations and skills. The clinical nurse educator must also be aware of academic policies that specify clinical learning expectations, behaviors of students, and skills that students can perform. Examples of policies from the practice environment that should be reviewed include needle stick or other injuries, specific skills that the student can or cannot perform, and instructions if a student commits a safety or judgment error.

Clinical nurse educators should understand the academic institution mission, philosophy, goals, policies, procedures, and course expectations to effectively blend academia with clinical learning and produce the desired outcomes. As discussed previously, Heshmati-Nabavi and Vanaki's (2010) grounded theory research, designed to understand perceptions of effective clinical nurse educators in Iran, reveals the theme of metacognition. A subcategory of this theme is knowledge of the curriculum. Gazza and Shellenbarger (2010) conducted a hermeneutic phenomenological study with nine clinical nurse educators to gain insight into the perspectives of part-time faculty members. They found that these part-time educators saw themselves as having limited information about the theory component of a nursing course and inadequate communication from the academic institution. Despite their clinical expertise, these educators had gaps in their understanding of the academic environment. Clinical nurse educators utilize clinical expertise when teaching by applying contemporary knowledge and understanding of client care to the clinical learning environment. Therefore, knowledge of the nursing school curricula and academic environment is essential.

To successfully navigate in the dual environments, clinical experts transitioning into the clinical nurse educator role need adequate preparation. They face numerous demands as they straddle the academic and practice settings. The process of embracing the role of the clinical nurse educator is a transformative journey that builds upon clinical expertise while merging with the academic environment and culture. The clinical nurse educator must navigate both worlds and follow policies and guidelines of both the practice and academic institutions to be successful.

IDENTIFIED GAPS IN THE LITERATURE

The articles reviewed for this analysis clearly indicate that a clinical nurse educator should be a clinical expert and possess clinical expertise; however, gaps were noted related to the role description. Although having clinical competence or practice expertise is frequently mentioned in various nursing education studies, the description of clinical expertise is rather superficial. Even in the qualitative studies, which are typically known for their rich descriptive narratives, the explanation about clinical expertise competencies and related task statements is scant.

Roberts et al. (2013), for example, used a naturalistic inquiry method to understand how clinical nurse educators describe their role and identify what may be missing for role actualization. The study, with 21 current or former adjunct faculty, does not provide foundational competencies for clinical nurses to be considered for the educator role, and this may be considered a gap. The study states that clinical nurses are being recruited by nursing programs for an educator role after one to several years of experience, but experience in the clinical practice environment can vary significantly. There is no universal list of competencies that clinical nurses need to achieve to be considered for a clinical nurse educator role.

Hou et al. (2011) conducted an exploratory factor analysis in China to develop and test psychometric properties of the Clinical Nursing Faculty Competence Inventory. This study, which looked at competency statements for the clinical nurse educator role, was one of the few quantitative studies reviewed. Participants included full-time nurse faculty, clinical nursing instructors, nursing education administrators, and undergraduate students. Competency statements included the following: proficiency in professional knowledge, identify trend and focus of nursing science development, confidence in professional knowledge and competence, reliable judgments and treatment according to clinical assessment, and proficiency in nursing research. The competencies identified in this study could be developed into a competency assessment for schools of nursing to use when interviewing potential clinical educators.

Heshmati-Nabavi and Vanaki (2010) performed a grounded theory research study in a baccalaureate nursing education program in Iran to identify nursing students and faculty members' perceptions of effective clinical nurse educator characteristics. They found five categories of effective clinical nurse educators: personal traits, metacognition, making clinical learning enjoyable, being a source of support, and being a role model. Subcategories associated with clinical expertise include knowledge of the clinical environment, turning theory into practice, clinical reasoning, and clinical competency. These subcategories are similar to clinical expert characteristics found in literature from the United States and other countries; however, the characteristics are not quantifiable. For example, this research states that "effective nursing educators are those who have sufficient experience gained in clinical settings" (p. 165). A gap exists related to what sufficient experience really means.

Andrew et al. (2010) performed semistructured interviews with sessional teachers in an undergraduate bachelor of nursing program in Australia. The researchers found that participants perceived the primary values that they brought to the clinical educator role were clinical currency, knowledge of the contemporary workplace, and experiential knowledge, but these concepts were not defined or measured, leading to ambiguity. The researchers stated that "sessional teachers in this study perceived an important aspect of their teaching was to bring the 'real' world of nursing to the classroom and to prepare students for the 'reality' of clinical practice" (p. 456). But this statement highlights important gaps: What is the real world of nursing, and how does it compare and contrast with classroom content and theory? What is the gap between theory and practice, and how should this gap be addressed from a research perspective?

The literature related to clinical expertise does not address other professional issues such as ethics, leadership, or evidence-based practices. When ethical dilemmas related to client care arise in the clinical learning environment, the clinical nurse educator must be equipped with tools and resources to assist students in processing the situation and applying the American Nurses Association (2015) *Code of Ethics for Nurses With Interpretive Statements*. The clinical nurse educator must be able to effectively guide students through tricky and often complicated dilemmas.

Additional components of the clinical expertise competency and task statements not found in research include knowledge of quality improvement, risk management, and legal considerations. Yet books related to clinical teaching often include information on these topics, suggesting the critical nature of these items (Fressola & Patterson, 2017; Gaberson et al., 2015; O'Connor, 2015; Oermann, 2015). This information should be included in a comprehensive orientation to the clinical learning environment to ensure that clinical nurse educators can navigate each topic in the academic and practice environments.

Given the continued explosion of technology in academia and health care, it should be noted that another gap evident in the literature relates to technology. Huston (2013) described the following emerging technologies that are transforming nursing practice: genetics and genomics, less invasive and more accurate tools for diagnosis and treatment, 3-D printing, robotics, biometrics, electronic health records, and computerized physician/provider order entry and clinical decision support. The author goes on to explain how clinical nurse skill sets must evolve to effectively provide client care, which would include skill sets of the clinical nurse educator. Concepts such as informatics and the use of technology and social media in the clinical learning environment should be considered.

Davidson and Rourke (2012) discuss the importance of understanding how to access and use an academic institution's website and intranet, university email, instructional software, and simulation equipment, but this represents only one aspect of technology knowledge necessary for the clinical nurse educator. They fail to discuss technology in the practice setting or clinical learning environment. With the emergence of technology and informatics in health care (e.g., electronic health records, bar code-scanned medications), the clinical nurse educator must learn about such technologies and use them in teaching. Duffy et al. (2008) also state the importance of clinical nurse educators using education technology to access course material and resources, but they do not discuss technology in the clinical learning environment. In addition, Hou et al. (2011) assessed clinical nurse educators for the ability to apply modern education technology to facilitate teaching. However, they do not address the ability to use technology in the clinical learning environment. This will continue to be a widening problem as technology further infiltrates health care delivery.

The breadth and depth of research in the area of clinical expertise in the clinical nurse educator role is lacking. Studies are primarily conducted at single sites using convenience samples and descriptive methodology, thus leading to concerns about generalizability. Additionally, little attention is focused on community-based clinical settings and graduate nursing education. Gaps in the research literature related to the clinical expertise competency and task statements provide fertile topics for additional study. The reviewed research lacks detailed and descriptive information about the influence of the practice setting, clinical learning environment, specialty areas, and other personal and professional variables that might influence the clinical expertise of the clinical nurse educator. It is unclear how these variables and the specific quantity and quality of each variable may influence the effectiveness of clinical nurse educators as they teach in the clinical learning environment.

PRIORITIES FOR FUTURE RESEARCH

Based upon the review of the literature, the following research priorities were identified and can be used to develop research questions to explore and better understand the clinical nurse educator competency of applying clinical expertise in the health care environment:

> What is the operational definition of clinical expertise?

> How could a concept analysis help to clarify and quantify the concept of clinical expertise?

> What specific components of clinical expertise are needed for success in the clinical nurse educator role? Do components differ for various clinical learning environments and level of the student?

> How do select professional practice environments such as specialty practice areas and practice settings impact the level of clinical expertise needed for effective teaching?

> What are foundational technology competencies for the clinical nurse educator role, and how should ongoing competency be assessed and measured?

> What are the characteristics of the transition to practice period for a clinical nurse educator to the clinical learning environment, and how does clinical expertise influence the transition period?

> How do clinical nurse educators integrate clinical expertise, best practices, and standards of care into the clinical learning environment?

> What makes up the gap between academic theory and clinical practice, and how should this gap be addressed from an evidence-based research perspective?

References

American Nurses Association. (2015). *Code of ethics for nurses with interpretive statements*. Silver Spring, MD: Author.

Andrew, S., Halcomb, E. J., Jackson, D., Peters, K., & Salamonson, Y. (2010). Sessional teachers in a BN program: Bridging the divide or widening the gap? *Nurse Education Today, 30*(5), 453–457. doi:10.1016/j.nedt.2009.10.004

Cangelosi, P., Crocker, S., & Sorrell, J. (2009). Expert to novice: Clinicians learning new roles as clinical nurse educators. *Nursing Education Perspectives, 30*(6), 367–371.

Dahlke, S., Baumbusch, J., Affleck, F., & Kwon, J. (2012). The clinical instructor role in nursing education: A structured literature review. *Journal of Nursing Education, 51*(12), 692–696. doi:10.3928/01484834-20121022-01

Davidson, K. M., & Rourke, L. (2012). Surveying the orientation learning needs of clinical nursing instructors. *International Journal of Nursing Education Scholarship, 9*(1), 1–11. doi:10.1515/1548-923X.2314

Duffy, N., Stuart, G., & Smith, S. (2008). Assuring the success of part-time faculty. *Nurse Educator, 33*(2), 53–54.

Esmaeili, M., Cheraghi, M. A., Salsali, M., & Ghiyasvandian, S. (2014). Nursing students' expectations regarding effective clinical education: A qualitative study. *International Journal of Nursing Practice, 20*(5), 460–467. doi:10.1111/ijn.12159

Flood, L. S., & Robinia, K. (2014). Bridging the gap: Strategies to integrate classroom and clinical learning. *Nurse Education in Practice, 14*(4), 329–332. doi:10.1016/j.nepr.2014.02.002

Fressola, M. C., & Patterson, G. E. (2017). *Transition from clinician to educator: A practical approach*. Burlington, MA: Jones & Bartlett.

Gaberson, K., Oermann, M., & Shellenbarger, T. (2015). *Clinical teaching strategies in nursing*. New York, NY: Springer.

Gazza, E. A., & Shellenbarger, T. (2010). The lived experience of part-time baccalaureate nursing faculty. *Journal of Professional Nursing, 26*(6), 353–359. doi:10.1016/j.profnurs.2010.08.002

Girija, K. (2012). Effective clinical instructor: A step toward excellence in clinical teaching. *International Journal of Nursing Education, 4*(1), 25–27.

Hall, N., & Chichester, M. (2014). How to succeed as an adjunct clinical nurse instructor. *Nursing for Women's Health, 18*(4), 341–344. doi:10.1111/1751-486X.12139

Hanson, K. J., & Stenvig, T. E. (2008). The good clinical nursing education and the baccalaureate nursing clinical experience: Attributes and praxis. *Journal of Nursing Education, 47*(1), 38–42.

Heshmati-Nabavi, F., & Vanaki, Z. (2010). Professional approach: The key feature of effective clinical educator in Iran. *Nurse Education Today, 30*(2), 163–168. doi:10.1016/j.nedt.2009.07.010

Hewitt, P., & Lewallen, L. (2010). Ready, set, teach! How to transform the clinical nurse expert into the part-time clinical nurse instructor. *Journal of Continuing Education in Nursing, 41*(9), 403–407.

Hou, X., Zhu, D., & Zheng, M. (2011). Clinical Nursing Faculty Competence Inventory—development and psychometric testing. *Journal of Advanced Nursing, 67*(5), 1109–1117. doi:10.1111.j.1365-2648.2010.05520.x

Hunt, C. W., Curtis, A. M., & Sanderson, B. K. (2013). A program to provide resources and support for clinical associates. *Journal of Continuing Education in Nursing, 44*(6), 269–273. doi:10.3928/00220124-20130402-27

Huston, C., (2013). The impact of emerging technology on nursing care: Warp speed ahead. *Online Journal of Issues in Nursing, 18*(2). doi: 10.3912/OJIN.Vol18No02Man01

Janzen, K. J. (2010). Alice through the looking glass: The influence of self and student understanding on role actualization among novice clinical nurse educators. *Journal of Continuing Education in Nursing, 41*(11), 517–523. doi:10.3928/00220124-20100701-07

Koharchik, L., & Jakub, K. (2014). Starting a job as adjunct clinical instructor. *American Journal of Nursing, 114*(8), 57–60. doi:10.1097/01.NAJ.0000453049.54489.d2

Kring, D. L., Ramseur, N., & Parnell, E. (2013). How effective are hospital adjunct clinical instructors? *Nursing Education Perspectives, 34*(1), 34–36.

O'Connor, A. B. (2015). *Clinical instruction and evaluation.* Burlington, MA: Jones & Bartlett.

Oermann, M. H. (2015). *Teaching in nursing and role of the educator: The complete guide to best practice in teaching, evaluation, and curriculum development.* New York, NY: Springer.

Peters, M. A., & Boylston, M. (2006). Mentoring adjunct faculty: Innovative solutions. *Nurse Educator, 31*(2), 61–64.

Poindexter, K. (2013). Novice nurse educator entry-level competency to teach: A national study. *Journal of Nursing Education, 52*(10), 559–566. doi:10.3928/01484834-20130913-04

Reid, T. P., Hinderer, K. A., Jarosinski, J. M., Mister, B. J., & Seldomridge, L. A. (2013). Expert clinician to clinical teacher: Developing a faculty academy and mentoring initiative. *Nurse Education in Practice, 13*(4), 288–293. doi:10.1016/j.nepr.2013.03.022

Roberts, K. K., Chrisman, S. K., & Flowers, C. (2013). The perceived needs of nurse clinicians as they move into an adjunct clinical faculty role. *Journal of Professional Nursing, 29*(5), 295–301. doi:10.1016/j.profnurs.2012.10.012

Robinson, C. P. (2009). Teaching and clinical educator competency: Bringing two worlds together. *International Journal of Nursing Education Scholarship, 6*(1), 1–14.

Santisteban, L., & Egues, A. L. (2014). Cultivating adjunct faculty: Strategies beyond orientation. *Nursing Forum, 49*(3), 152–158.

Volk, S., Homan, N., Tepner, L., Chichester, M., & Scales, D. (2013). The rewards and challenges of becoming a clinical instructor. *Nursing for Women's Health, 17*(6), 539–542. doi:10.1111/1751-486X.12083

West, M., Borden, C., Bermudez, M., Hanson-Zalot, M., Amorim, F., & Marmion, R. (2009). Enhancing the clinical adjunct role to benefit students. *Journal of Continuing Education in Nursing, 40*(7), 305–310. doi:10.3928/00220124-20090623-05

Wiens, S., Babenko-Mould, Y., & Iwasiw, C. (2014). Clinical instructors' perceptions of structured and psychological empowerment in academic nursing environments. *Journal of Nursing Education, 53*(5), 265–270. doi:10.3928/01484834-20140421-01

6

Facilitate Learner Development and Socialization

Teresa Shellenbarger, PhD, RN, CNE, ANEF
Wanda Bonnel, PhD, APRN, ANEF

Clinical nurse educators create an environment that facilitates learner development and socializes students to the professional nursing role. Like the academic nurse educator, clinical nurse educators recognize their responsibility for helping students develop as nurses and integrate the values and behaviors expected of those who fulfill that role (National League for Nursing [NLN], 2012b). During clinical learning experiences, the clinical nurse educator helps students learn about professional nursing behaviors, standards, and ethical principles that guide practice. Through mentoring and modeling, they create an environment conducive to helping learners develop and become socialized to the nursing role.

The following task statements include the knowledge, skills, and attitudes that clinical nurse educators must develop to *facilitate learner development and socialization.* The clinical nurse educator:

- Mentors learners in the development of professional nursing behaviors, standards, and codes of ethics
- Promotes a learning climate of respect for all
- Promotes professional integrity and accountability
- Maintains professional boundaries
- Encourages ongoing learner professional development via formal and informal venues
- Assists learners in effective use of self-assessment and professional goal setting for ongoing self-improvement
- Creates learning environments that are focused on socialization to the role of the nurse
- Assists learners to develop the ability to engage in constructive peer feedback

> Inspires creativity and confidence
> Encourages various techniques to manage stress (e.g., relaxation, meditation, mindfulness)
> Role models self-reflection, self-care, and coping skills
> Empowers learners to be successful in meeting professional and educational goals
> Engages learners in applying best practices and quality improvement processes.

REVIEW OF THE LITERATURE

A review of the nursing and related literature for this competency, including the 13 task statements, revealed limited research. Several national studies were available; however, research was primarily based on single-site, small-scale research studies relevant to facilitating learner development and socialization. This review draws from larger national studies and professional publications that are commonly endorsed in nursing and nursing education. Two major themes emerged from this literature focusing on facilitating learner development and socialization. Those themes are supporting professional identity formation and serving as a professional role model.

Supporting Professional Identity Formation

The first theme that emerged in this literature involves supporting student socialization to the profession and guiding students in their development of a nursing identity. Clinical nurse educators use a variety of strategies to support students in their enculturation into nursing so that they can learn to function effectively as a nurse. They empower learners to reach their educational and professional goals; internalize the nursing culture; and acquire professional knowledge, skills, and attitudes needed to function in the changing health care environment. Clinical nurse educators have the opportunity to change students' perspectives as they learn about the profession and build their knowledge and confidence so that they are adequately prepared for future work. Although limited research exists that elaborates on this process, some references do provide a beginning glimpse into the strategies that clinical nurse educators use in guiding students toward professional behaviors.

Students need to understand and operate under the rules, expectations, norms, and culture that guide professional behavior. Clinical nurse educators use standards, codes, and guidelines to direct nursing actions. Knowing how to behave as a professional is directed by regularly updated professional documents such as the American Nurses Association (ANA) *Code of Ethics for Nurses With Interpretive Statements* (ANA, 2015a) and *Nursing: Scope and Standards of Nursing Practice* (ANA, 2015b), other professional documents developed by national nursing organizations, and other relevant publications for individual nursing specialties. These essential documents provide a useful guide for nursing and nursing education. Morin (2015), for example, described the ANA *Code of Ethics for Nurses* as relevant and important in today's rapidly changing health care environment. She noted a multitude of current and emerging topics, such as social media use, incivility, end-of-life issues, genetic engineering, and the changing health care environment, as examples of timely topics that may present ethical dilemmas that nurses, educators, and students face.

Given the challenging clinical situations confronting nurses in health care today, the ANA *Code of Ethics for Nurses With Interpretive Statements* (ANA, 2015a), which is frequently used to guide clinical nursing decisions, underwent a rigorous revision process to remain current. The recent revision involved more than 2,700 public comments suggesting the need for revisions, the creation of a 15-member steering committee to draft revisions, and an opportunity for public comment. Nearly 1,000 individuals provided input that was then analyzed and used to inform the final version of the document (Epstein & Turner, 2015). Although this process did not specifically focus on clinical nurse educators, the resulting code created by this group clearly impacts clinical nurse educators and their teaching. It offers a guide for decision-making by clinical nurse educators and students when confronted with ethical dilemmas in the clinical learning environment.

Other professional organizations, such as the National League for Nursing (NLN), have recognized that nurse educators may face other complex and challenging ethical issues in their teaching role. To further clarify ethical situations faced by nurse educators, the NLN provided additional guidance by publishing *Ethical Principles for Nursing Education* (NLN, 2012a). Although this document is not based on a single research study, it was informed by sound knowledge of health care, practice, and educational issues. It serves as an essential guide for clinical nurse educators.

Not only must nurses, nurse educators, and students contend with ethical issues, but the profession is also faced with changes in the health care system that lead to ethical dilemmas. These changes are creating a growing demand for nurses at a time when the United States is experiencing a shortage of nurses and nurse educators. The Carnegie Foundation for the Advancement of Teaching was concerned with how professionals such as nurses are prepared given these changes. They supported a landmark multiyear comparative study of professional education and included nursing as part of the professional practice preparation study. Benner, Sutphen, Leonard, and Day (2010) report on their extensive field research conducted at nine diverse nursing schools offering nursing education across the spectrum of educational programs (prelicensure through master entry-level programs). The second phase of their research involved national surveys conducted in collaboration with leading national nursing organizations. Select study highlights are relevant to the theme of supporting socialization, specifically what they refer to as "ethical comportment" or the "incalculation, infusion, or instantiation of the responsibilities, concerns, and commitments of the profession" (Day, Benner, Sutphen, & Leonard, 2009, p. 74). Their study revealed that ethical issues are embedded in student clinical practice and equated with nursing practice. Nursing programs and clinical nurse educators introduce students to ethical comportment and professional values during their clinical learning situations. Benner et al. (2010) recommend that nurse educators intentionally provide opportunities through experiential learning, such as in clinical settings, to create the formation of professional identity and not just socialization to the role.

Reflection has been described as a tool to help deal with ethical issues and other challenges that students may face in the clinical setting. Reflection is well documented as an evidence-based practice that provides an opportunity for students to think about their experiences and to learn from them (Horton-Deutsch, Sherwood, & Armstrong, 2012). Using reflection as part of clinical teaching and learning can help students understand the underlying meaning of experiences. Reflective activities may help students as they transform from a novice learner and begin to assume the identity of a professional nurse. As noted, reflective activities can also be a component of ongoing assessment, self-improvement, and professional development. Clinical nurse educators can assist learners to engage in thoughtful and constructive self-evaluative activities by incorporating reflection opportunities in their clinical teaching (Horton-Deutsch et al., 2012).

Numerous studies conducted by nurse educators have used reflective activities to promote learning about nursing and the profession. Ganzer and Zauderer (2013) found that a structured preclinical workshop on common mental health issues and therapeutic communication, combined with self-reflection, was useful in helping 30 baccalaureate nursing students increase self-awareness and decrease anxiety during a psychiatric/mental health clinical experience. Reflection, in the form of reflective learning journals, has also been used to enhance student learning outcomes, including a study of 32 students enrolled in an online graduate nursing education course (Langley & Brown, 2010). Even though the course did not involve clinical learning, the student perceptions of improved learning and notation of challenges to reflective journaling are still important in helping educators understand how reflective learning journals can help students develop as professionals and may be applicable for clinical nurse educators. Another study of 39 associate degree nursing students, conducted by Van Horn and Freed (2008), employed reflective journaling with guided questions and dialogue pairs to solve clinical problems. Qualitative data analysis revealed that the use of these reflection strategies led to increases in reflection during the study period. These authors also found that these reflective journals enabled students to connect their clinical experiences to previous experiences or to classroom learning and promoted learning.

Another important aspect of professional identity formation that emerges from clinical nursing education involves caring and demonstrating respect for others. Students need to learn and practice respect for others and address issues related to diversity. Nursing students can learn about these concepts in the classroom, but they become real for them when encountered in the clinical learning environment. Clinical nurse educators provide opportunities for students to acquire and practice these components of nursing professional identity in the clinical setting. While guiding nursing care by students in the clinical setting, clinical nurse educators model caring and inclusive behaviors. This education begins with the clinical nurse educator demonstrating respect for students, patients, and others in the health care setting. The need for demonstration of respect by clinical nurse educators is supported in research by Klunklin et al. (2011). Using the Self-Evaluation Scale on Role Modeling Behaviors with 320 nursing faculty from four nursing schools in Thailand, they found that clinical nurse educators reported encouraging an atmosphere of mutual respect with this behavior emerging as the highest rated item in the study. The authors speculate that clinical nurse educators' demonstration of respect, empathy, and student support encourages mutual respect.

Establishing a climate of respect for others happens with the use of appropriate, clear communication, which then sets the stage for ongoing professional development. Concepts related to respectful clinical nurse educator communication that are discussed in the literature include using open interpersonal communication that is encouraging, cooperative, friendly, and supportive rather than discouraging (Esmaeili, Cheraghi, Salsali, & Ghiyasvandian, 2014; Girija, 2012). Offering constructive feedback, providing clear direction, and sharing expectations are other effective approaches to communicate professional experiences and attitudes (Hanson & Stenvig, 2008; Hossein, Fatemeh, Fatemeh, Katri, & Tahereh, 2010). Research conducted by Esmaeili et al. (2014) concurs. Participants in this qualitative study of 17 Iranian nursing students were interviewed and asked to describe effective clinical education. The researchers found that effective and appropriate communication between clinical nurse educators and students was among the most important expectations that students had for effective clinical education. The authors further elaborate and suggest that good communication, which creates a sense of trust, is critical to illustrate appropriate behavior and modeling of professionalism for students.

Serving as a Professional Role Model

A second theme emerging from the literature, related to facilitating learner development and socialization, involves professional role modeling. Students observe the attitudes and actions of the clinical nurse educator and frequently model or imitate what they see. Thus, when faculty demonstrate personal and professional qualities such as compassion, integrity, and honesty when delivering quality, evidence-based, ethical and legally correct care, students notice and may emulate the behaviors they see.

It has been suggested that clinical nurse educators are "professional role models for students and are responsible for creating learning environments that socialize students into the profession" (Halstead, 2009, p. 137). This is further described in a qualitative study using interviews of 10 students and clinical educators to determine perceptions of effective clinical educator characteristics. Relevant to role modeling, one of the five significant categories emerging from the data, one participant stated, "I think the clinical educator has to be a role model. We can envisage 'a good nurse'" (Heshmati-Nabavi & Vanaki, 2010, p. 166). Students observing faculty demonstrating appropriate nursing care can gain information from this powerful role modeling approach to professional behavior. Learning by observation can be further enhanced by reflective activities such as journaling or group discussions. Students have an opportunity to think critically about what they have witnessed, consider the knowledge gained, and ponder the implications of the actions.

When clinical nurse educators teach by example, students in the clinical setting can learn about professional nursing from these role models. Some researchers address the importance of role modeling in their publications about clinical nurse educators (Hossein et al., 2010; Hou, Zhu, & Zheng, 2011; Poindexter, 2013). Hossein et al. (2010), in interviews with 15 nursing teachers in Iran, found that one theme was multiplicity in teaching style. A component of that theme involved teaching by being a role model. Interviews revealed that "nursing teachers believed that being a role model in clinical education is the most effective and right way for transmitting professional experiences and attitudes" (p. 10). The clinical nurse educator transmits the right attitudes about nursing and the fulfillment of professional responsibilities. This suggests that even if clinical educators believe they are only demonstrating actions and not providing explanations, students are still being socialized and learning about the professional nursing role through the examples they see. These conclusions are further supported by findings from the Poindexter (2013) study, which sought to identify nursing education competencies by surveying 374 nursing program administrators from 48 states in the United States. Findings from this national sample reveal an expectation across all institution types that nurse educators facilitate professional socialization. In a study by Hou et al. (2011), clinical managers, educators, and students unanimously agreed that fostering nursing student professional growth was a top item of importance.

Professional role modeling by clinical nurse educators occurs beyond patient care delivery and is evident in other professional activities that may be observed by the nursing student. A profession is expected to have a body of knowledge that guides practice. Nursing has this specialized knowledge base, but nursing professionals struggle to remain up-to-date given the rapid development of new knowledge that impacts practice. Nursing professionals need to remain abreast of current professional developments. As noted by an influential Institute of Medicine (IOM) report (2011), *The Future of Nursing: Leading Change, Advancing Health,* lifelong learning is a key component to self-improvement and practice. "The committee recommends that nurses and nursing students and faculty continue their education and engage in lifelong learning" (IOM, 2011, p. 4). Participation in lifelong learning is modeled by clinical nurse educators and illustrates to students how continued development is essential for maintenance of competent practice. Professional development may focus on remaining up-to-date with evidence-based practices, engagement in quality improvement initiatives, and being knowledgeable about professional initiatives and new developments in patient care— all important areas to role model for students.

Robinson (2009), in her framework for evaluation of clinical educators, suggests that clinical nurse educators can role model professional behaviors by attending in-service educational programs, learning new policies and procedures at the clinical facility, participating in continued learning via continuing education workshops and training, and belonging to professional organizations. The importance of role modeling ongoing professional development is also discussed in the descriptive study of nursing faculty members in Thailand by Klunklin et al. (2011). These authors recommend that clinical nurse educators demonstrate professional development by attending conferences and reading journals.

Modeling patient advocacy and policy development also empowers learners (Day et al., 2009). There is limited research specific to the clinical educator role in this arena; however, broader approaches include a qualitative study by Wiens, Babenko-Mould, and Iwasiw (2014). These authors interviewed eight clinical instructors to gain their perceptions of structural and psychological empowerment in their clinical teaching. Limited feedback and limited mentoring were noted to be common experiences. Although academic support and gaining confidence were noted as important, faculty indicated that further strategies to achieve empowerment as clinical educators are needed. To ensure that clinical nurse educators can perform effectively as role models and patient advocates, they need adequate ongoing support as they shift from clinical nursing to clinical teaching roles.

Another area that clinical nurse educators may need to enhance involves modeling for nursing students the delivery of safe, quality nursing care. In a summary of work of the Think Tank on Transforming Clinical Education, Armstrong, Sherwood, and Tagliareni (2009) address various national reports, including the Quality and Safety Education for Nurses (QSEN) project. Using surveys and focus groups, they found that students doubted that faculty held the needed expertise to teach quality and safety concepts. The authors identified the importance of reframing nursing education to focus on quality and safety as a key part of nursing education and professional identity formation.

Phase II of the QSEN project involved piloting and testing teaching strategies that would advance the QSEN competencies. Fifteen pilot nursing schools worked to develop quality and safety competencies in prelicensure nursing programs, with this work evolving into various faculty development initiatives (Bednash, Cronenwett, & Dolansky, 2013). These QSEN initiatives have led to many innovations in nursing education and clearly continue to influence clinical nurse education and the work of nurse educators.

Quality improvement activities and initiatives such as QSEN help students identify best evidence to promote safe, quality care. Tools and strategies can be used by clinical nurse educators to assess the ongoing use of best practices and identification of opportunities for practice improvements. Additional resources, such as QSEN and materials from the Institute for Healthcare Improvement (IHI), are being developed and can provide guidance to clinical nurse educators. However, further research about best practices for engaging students and role modeling these practices related to quality improvement is needed.

IDENTIFIED GAPS IN THE LITERATURE

Facilitating learner development and socialization to the professional role is a complex issue deserving further study. Discussion of this competency and task statements were organized by two major themes: supporting professional identity formation and serving as a professional role model. Research gaps are identified for each of these themes and provide opportunity for further study across all nursing education levels. Select needs and challenges related to this competency are documented by national studies and reports. Theory-based articles, national reports, and project descriptions are the most common evidence for this competency. Available research related to this competency is primarily based on single-site, small-scale research studies, but some national multisite, multimethod approaches are included. These research reports provide a foundation to begin clarifying the competencies and task statements, but further study is crucial. As noted by Ard and Valiga (2009), it is time to rethink the elements and models for clinical education. It is also important to move beyond descriptive and exploratory studies to comparative and experimental studies that can produce the strongest evidence to better understand the outcomes of interest and the effectiveness of interventions.

PRIORITIES FOR FUTURE RESEARCH

Based upon the review of the literature, the following research questions have been identified and can be used to stimulate research to enhance understanding of the clinical nurse educator competency of facilitating learning development and socialization. The following questions reflect priorities for future research:

- How do clinical nurse educators socialize students to the role of the professional nurse?

- What clinical educator strategies or approaches are the most effective in promoting learner socialization and identity formation?

- How can clinical partners best be engaged to promote or guide student socialization?

- What are the best strategies to facilitate values development in nursing students?

- What strategies are most effective in enhancing clinical educator role modeling for students? For example, does reflective journaling promote professional growth for clinical educators? For their students?

- What are best strategies for using national initiatives such as QSEN in preparing students for their professional roles? How can students be best guided in engaging patients as participants in safe, quality care?

References

American Nurses Association. (2015a). *Code of ethics for nurses with interpretive statements*. Silver Spring, MD: Author.

American Nurses Association. (2015b). *Nursing: Scope and standards of nursing practice*. Silver Spring, MD: Author.

Ard, N., & Valiga, T. (2009). *Clinical nursing education: Current reflections*. New York, NY: National League for Nursing.

Armstrong, G., Sherwood, G., & Tagliareni, M. E. (2009). Quality and safety education in nursing (QSEN): Integrating recommendations from IOM into clinical nursing education. In N. Ard & T. Valiga (Eds.), *Clinical nursing education: Current reflections*. (pp. 207–226). New York, NY: National League for Nursing.

Bednash, G. P., Cronenwett, L., & Dolansky, M. A. (2013). QSEN transforming education. *Journal of Professional Nursing, 29*(2), 66–67. doi:10.1016/j.profnurs.2013.03.001

Benner, P., Sutphen, M., Leonard, V., & Day, L. (2010). *Educating nurses: A call for radical transformation*. San Francisco, CA: Jossey-Bass.

Day, L., Benner, P., Sutphen, M., & Leonard, V. (2009). Reflections on clinical education: Insights from the Carnegie Study. In N. Ard, & T. Valiga (Eds.), *Clinical nursing education: Current reflections*. (pp. 71–90). New York, NY: National League for Nursing.

Epstein, B., & Turner, M. (2015). The nursing code of ethics: Its values, its history. *OJIN: The Online Journal of Issues in Nursing, 20*(2). doi:10.3912/OJIN.Vol2No02Man04

Esmaeili, M., Cheraghi, M. A., Salsali, M., & Ghiyasvandian, S. (2014). Nursing students' expectations regarding effective clinical education: A qualitative study. *International Journal of Nursing Practice, 20*(5), 460–467. doi:10.1111/ijn.12159

Ganzer, C. A., & Zauderer, C. (2013). Structured learning and self-reflection: Strategies to decrease anxiety in the psychiatric mental health clinical nursing experience. *Nursing Education Perspectives, 34*(4), 244–247.

Girija, K. M. (2012). Effective clinical instructor: A step toward excellence in clinical teaching. *International Journal of Nursing Education, 4*(1), 25–27.

Halstead, J. (2009) Reflections on clinical education: Insights from the Carnegie Study. In N. Ard, & T. Valiga (Eds.), *Clinical nursing education: Current reflections* (pp. 133–144). New York, NY: National League for Nursing.

Hanson, K. J., & Stenvig, T. E. (2008). The good clinical nursing educator and the baccalaureate nursing clinical experience: Attributes and praxis. *Journal of Nursing Education, 47*(1), 38–42.

Heshmati-Nabavi, F., & Vanaki, Z. (2010). Professional approach: The key feature of effective clinical educator in Iran. *Nurse Education Today, 30*(2), 163–168. doi:10.1016/j.nedt.2009.07.010

Horton-Deutsch, S., Sherwood, G., & Armstrong, G. (2012). Reflection in classroom and clinical contexts: Assessment and evaluation. In G. Sherwood & S. Horton-Deutsch (Eds.), *Transforming education and improving outcomes* (pp. 169–186). Indianapolis, IN: Sigma Theta Tau International.

Hossein, K. M., Fatemeh, D., Fatemeh, O. S., Katri, V., & Tahereh, B. (2010). Teaching style in clinical nursing education: A qualitative study of Iranian nursing teacher's experiences. *Nurse Education in Practice, 10*(1), 8–12. doi:10.1016/j.nepr.2009.01.016

Hou, X., Zhu, D., & Zheng, M. (2011). Clinical Nursing Faculty Competence Inventory—development and psychometric testing. *Journal of Advanced Nursing, 67*(5), 1109–1117. doi:10.1111/j.1365-2648.2010.05520.x

Institute of Medicine. (2011). *The future of nursing: Leading change, advancing health.* Washington, DC: National Academies Press.

Klunklin, A., Sawasdisingha, P., Viserkul, N., Fusnashima, N., Kameoka, T., Nomoto, Y., & Nakayama, T. (2011). Role model behaviors of nursing faculty members in Thailand. *Nursing and Health Sciences, 13*(1), 84–87. doi:10.1111/j.1442-2018.2011.00585.x

Langley, M. E., & Brown, S. T. (2010). Perceptions of the use of reflection learning journals in online graduate nursing education. *Nursing Education Perspectives, 31*(1), 12–17.

Morin, K. (2015). The code of ethics for nurses—more relevant than ever. *Journal of Nursing Education, 54*(12), 667–668. doi:10.3928/01484834-20151110-01

National League for Nursing. (2012a). *Ethical principles for nursing education.* Retrieved from http://www.nln.org/docs/default-source/default-document-library/ethical-principles-for-nursing-education-final-final-010312.pdf?sfvrsn=z

National League for Nursing. (2012b). *The scope of practice for academic nurse educators.* New York, NY: Author.

Poindexter, K. (2013). Novice nurse educator entry-level competency to teach: A national study. *Journal of Nursing Education, 52*(10), 559–566. doi:10.3928/01484834-20130913-04

Robinson, C. P. (2009). Teaching and clinical educator competency: Bringing two worlds together. *International Journal of Nursing Education Scholarship, 6*(1), 1–14. doi:10.2202/1548-923X.1793

Van Horn, R., & Freed, S. (2008). Journaling and dialogue pairs to promote reflection in clinical nursing education. *Nursing Education Perspectives, 29*(4), 220–225.

Wiens, S., Babenko-Mould, Y., & Iwasiw, C. (2014). Clinical instructors' perceptions of structural and psychological empowerment in academic nursing environments. *Journal of Nursing Education, 53*(5), 265–270. doi:10.3928/01484834-20140421-01

7

Implement Effective Clinical Assessment and Evaluation Strategies

Amber M. Patrick, PhD, RN, CNE, COI

Clinical nurse educators have a unique opportunity to provide direct assessment and evaluation of learners in the clinical learning environment. Given small instructor-to-learner ratios and the time spent in one-on-one contact with learners in the clinical laboratory, simulation, and/or clinical setting, the clinical nurse educator is in an ideal position to observe clinical performance and make evaluative decisions. However, educators across all levels and program types may struggle to effectively assess and evaluate students consistently. Outcomes of student learning and performance expectations may not be clear, and the dynamic nature of the clinical setting compounds concerns that clinical nurse educators face regarding assessment and evaluation. Additionally, the evaluation process involves the measurement of multiple dimensions of practice. Given the impact of evaluation, it is an emotionally charged activity (Hewitt & Lewallen, 2010). Learners and educators would benefit from clarity regarding these evaluation issues so that clinical nurse educator efforts can focus on the achievement of learner outcomes and progression to safe, competent nursing practice.

This competency and the following 11 task statements include the knowledge, skills, and attitudes that clinical nurse educators must develop to *implement effective clinical assessment and evaluation strategies*. The clinical nurse educator:

➤ Uses a variety of assessment and evaluation strategies to determine achievement of learning outcomes

➤ Implements both formative and summative evaluation that is appropriate to the learner and learning outcomes

➤ Engages in timely communication with course faculty regarding learner clinical performance

➤ Maintains integrity in the assessment and evaluation of learners

➤ Provides timely, objective, constructive, and fair feedback to learners

> Uses assessment and evaluation data to enhance the teaching-learning process in the clinical learning environment
> Demonstrates skill in the use of best practices in the assessment and evaluation of clinical performance
> Assesses and evaluates appropriate clinical performance expectations
> Assesses learner strengths and weaknesses in the clinical learning environment using performance standards
> Documents learner clinical performance, feedback, and progression
> Evaluates the quality of clinical learning experiences and the environment.

REVIEW OF THE LITERATURE

A review of the nursing and related literature revealed limited evidence-based research related to assessment and evaluation strategies in clinical nursing education and the 11 associated task statements. Many clinical nurse educators receive insufficient preparation to confront the challenges of assessment and evaluation. They may rely on their own clinical expertise or past experiences to measure learner outcome achievement instead of relying on evidence-based assessment and evaluation strategies (Clark, Alcala-Van Houten, & Perea-Ryan, 2010; Dattilo, Brewer, & Streit, 2009; Hemman, Gillingham, Allison, & Adams, 2007). Research to validate the effectiveness of clinical assessment and evaluation strategies employed by clinical nurse educators is lacking in the current literature. The following discussion characterizes the themes identified from the research literature, scholarly books, and articles related to the effective implementation of assessment and evaluation strategies by clinical nurse educators. These themes are assessment and evaluation of learning outcomes in the clinical learning environment, and assessment and evaluation strategies. The literature associated with these themes is discussed in the following section of this chapter.

The purpose of clinical assessment and evaluation is to provide data about the knowledge, skills, and attitudes required of students as they relate to an established standard of care (Bonnel, 2016). To conduct effective and accurate clinical assessment and evaluation, clinical nurse educators must first reflect on their own values and biases related to assessment and evaluation, ensure that they base evaluation on established outcomes using appropriate methods and tools, and promote an encouraging clinical learning environment that will foster student success (Gaberson, Oermann, & Shellenbarger, 2015).

Assessment and Evaluation of Learning Outcomes in the Clinical Learning Environment

It is imperative that the clinical outcomes evaluated by clinical nurse educators are consistent with the fundamental outcomes required for nursing degree acquisition. As noted by Holaday and Buckley (2008), inconsistent clinical assessment and evaluation is associated with insufficient preparation of nurse graduates. By reducing the educational variations between clinical competencies and essential learning outcomes, clinical nurse educators can better ensure that nurse graduates are equipped with the skills and knowledge needed to practice as safe and competent health care professionals. In 2003, the Institute of Medicine (IOM) called for changes in health professional education, including a focus on competency- or outcome-based assessment. The IOM recommended five core competencies that all health care providers, including nurses, should demonstrate: demonstration of patient-centered care, interdisciplinary team care, use of evidence-based practice, quality improvement practices, and utilization of informatics (Greiner & Knebel, 2003). Competencies in these crucial areas are necessary in assessing learning, as they undergird the evaluation of learning outcomes and clearly outline the skills, knowledge, behaviors, and values that should be developed over time (Sullivan, 2016). However, the mere establishment of outcomes is not enough. The knowledge, skills, and attitudes supporting each outcome should be clearly communicated and associated measures of assessment established by the clinical nurse educator. Assessment tools should be relevant to the outcomes being assessed, and results should show evidence that goals and objectives have been met. Effective assessment and evaluation strategies linked to learning outcomes are discussed in the next section.

Clinical experiences provide an opportunity for students to transfer what is learned in the classroom, simulations, readings, and other experiences to their care for patients. In clinical practice, students face complex, multidimensional problems that are not always easily solved with scientific theory and thinking. When faced with such problems, students learn to develop their critical thinking and clinical judgment skills—both essential outcomes for nurse graduates (Oermann & Gaberson, 2017).

Assessment and evaluation of learning outcomes in the clinical learning environment can be challenging for clinical nurse educators when critical thinking, problem solving, and clinical judgment are factors that affect the achievement of specific competencies. Additionally, with clinical learning environments being fast paced and often unpredictable, objectives and outcomes must serve as a learning guide. Clinical nurse educators must be able to offer useful and constructive feedback to promote clinical learning so that students can achieve the desired outcome and become competent nurses (Esmaeili, Cheraghi, Salsali, & Ghiyasvandian, 2014; Girija, 2012). Unfortunately, the literature suggests that not all clinical nurse educators are adequately prepared for these clinical evaluation and grading activities (Forbes, Hickey, & White, 2010).

To be clinically competent, the learner must use theoretical and clinical knowledge to provide appropriate patient care. Various approaches to measuring clinical competence have been studied. O'Connor, Fealy, Kelly, McGuinness, and Timmins (2009) describe the development of an evaluation tool that can be used by clinical nurse educators to assess the competence of nursing students. Development of the Shared Specialist Placement Document (SSPD), a criterion-referenced assessment tool, was based upon standards for nursing practice in Ireland. The tool was designed to be adaptable to a wide range of clinical experiences and settings. Use of the SSPD requires formal meetings between the student and clinical teacher and adequate documentation of student progression. The tool was tested with a convenience sample of 29 bachelor degree nursing students and their preceptors ($n = 27$) from three universities in Ireland. Participants were satisfied with the assessment tool for clinical evaluation. O'Connor et al. (2009) report the highest positive correlations for students and clinical nurse educators to be the positive perceptions of the learning plan that is devised using the tool (preceptors $r = 0.839$, $p < .01$; students $r = 0.579$, $p < .01$). Open-ended qualitative findings suggest that clinical nurse educators need preparation and support for use of the tool, as well as adequate time to complete assessments.

Another clinical evaluation tool that reports psychometric testing and can be used by clinical nurse educators in both simulation and other clinical settings is the Quint Leveled Clinical Competency Tool (QLCCT). This tool measures prelicensure nursing students' clinical judgment by assessing 10 competencies at four possible levels (Prion, Gilbert, Adamson, Kardong-Edgren, & Quint, 2017). This tool was adapted from the Tanner (2006) model and reflects four developmental progressive levels of competence, moving from novice, progressing, advancing, to graduate nurse. The tool was tested over three phases in a multisite, multiyear study. "Preliminary psychometric testing demonstrates good interrater reliability (0.87), content validity index (0.72) and coefficient alpha (0.83)" (Prion et al., 2017, p. 106). Based upon these results, the QLCCT represents a suitable tool for clinical nurse educators to use for measurement of clinical competencies with simulation experiences and represents beginning work demonstrating a statistically supported evaluation tool.

Objective structured clinical examinations (OSCEs), using stations where students are required to demonstrate select nursing care, have also been used by clinical nurse educators to assess and evaluate clinical skill performance. OSCEs are becoming more widely accepted as a standardized evaluation approach even though validity and reliability are not always established or reported. One study that does report the development and psychometric testing of an OSCE was conducted by Selim, Ramadan, El-Gueneidy, and Gaafer (2012). They conclude that their OSCE, used with 76 Egyptian students in psychiatric nursing education, is a reliable and valid method of assessing clinical competency. They describe statistically significant positive correlations (agreement) between raters, with a Cronbach's alpha greater than 0.7 for 7 of 11 OSCE stations. They also report a statistically significant correlation between OSCE and other evaluation criteria, leading to the conclusion that this evaluation method is a valid and reliable approach for clinical outcome evaluation that can be used by clinical nurse educators.

The preceding findings are consistent with a previously published systematic review of undergraduate nursing student clinical assessment conducted by Wu, Enskär, Lee, and Wang (2015). Using the PRISMA checklist and the *Cochrane Handbook for Systematic Reviews of Interventions*, Wu et al. completed a review that examined current assessment practices of undergraduate nursing students for the period from 2000 to 2013. They reviewed 14 qualitative and quantitative research studies on this topic. Interestingly, all studies originated from countries outside the United States—Australia, Denmark, Germany, Ireland, Norway, Scotland, Sweden, Turkey, and Taiwan. The findings were the same as those identified previously in the literature. The researchers concluded that clinical nurse educators have concerns about evaluation practices due to insufficient evidence to substantiate reliability and validity of the assessment tools. They determined that many "studies ensured face and content validity of the assessment tool by obtaining consensus through discussion with nurse experts. However, most of the studies reported this process without statistical data to support the content validity test" (Wu et al., 2015, pp. 357–358). Wu et al. suggest that some tools are linked to criterion validity with outcomes associated with national nursing standards—a conclusion that remains true for the simulation literature as well.

This literature suggests that there are a few studies addressing outcomes assessment and evaluation of learning outcomes with psychometrically sound, reliable, and valid measurement tools for clinical nurse educator use. Although this is an important competency for clinical nurse educators to master, gaps remain in this literature that do not provide adequate evidence to direct clinical nurse educator practices regardless of the clinical site (Holaday & Buckley, 2008).

Assessment and Evaluation Strategies

The assessment and evaluation of clinical performance poses continued challenges for clinical nurse educators. Nurse educators have used a range of strategies to assess and evaluate students' clinical performance, but little evidence exists to show the effectiveness of these strategies. Observation, rubrics, questioning, written assignments, skills testing, simulation, self-reflection, and self-assessment are a few examples of assessment and evaluation strategies presented in the literature (McCarthy & Murphy, 2008; Oermann, Kardong-Edgren, & Rizzolo, 2016; Oermann, Saewert, Charasika, & Yarbrough, 2009a). The following section of this chapter discusses specific assessment and evaluation strategies that may be used by clinical nurse educators, including rubrics, observation, simulation, and OSCE.

Rubrics

Clinical evaluation is influenced in part by an evaluator's subjectivity and perspective (Oermann & Gaberson, 2017). For this reason, Stevens and Mattsson (2016) suggest that clinical nurse educators use rubrics to measure clinical performance of nursing students. Rubrics can help students and clinical nurse educators by decreasing confusion about expectations, provide evaluation criteria to gauge achievement, decrease subjectivity in the clinical evaluation process, promote evaluation transparency, and enhance communication.

Isaacson and Stacy (2009) discuss rubrics and describe the benefits of use by clinical nurse educators. They also discuss the development of rubrics for clinical assessment and evaluation in nursing, stating that rubrics "facilitate communication because feedback can be given quickly, fairly, efficiently, and individually" (p. 137). Rubrics could also be adapted to meet the needs of individual clinical courses and linked to course objectives. Additional benefits of rubrics include facilitating tracking of student progress over time, providing a platform to detail explicit communication to all involved in the assessment and evaluation process, and specifying a direct connection between clinical behavior and grades. The utilization of rubrics is one possible answer to clinical nurse educator concerns about clinical evaluation.

Another article further supports the use of rubrics as a clinical assessment and evaluation approach to assess the clinical performance of nursing students. Skúladóttir and Svavarsdóttir (2016) describe the development of the Clinical Assessment Tool for Nursing Education (CAT-NE) based upon mixed-method data collection in Iceland. The researchers used a variety of data collection approaches, including structured interviewing, discussion groups, and questionnaires, to develop the criterion-referenced CAT-NE. Through psychometric testing with clinical educators, clinical experts, RNs, and students, the researchers concluded that the CAT-NE offers a valid assessment tool for clinical assessment. Rubrics, such as those found on the CAT-NE, that use descriptive performance criteria allow clinical nurse educators to minimize subjectivity, improve the evaluation process, clarify expectations, and evaluate clinical performance with a valid tool.

An assessment tool developed by Ulfvarson and Oxelmark (2012) in Sweden provides clinical nurse educators with another assessment and evaluation strategy for the clinical learning environment. The authors report on the development and testing of the Assessment of Clinical Education (ACIEd) tool as part of an extensive, multistep development and validation process, with students, preceptors, practicing nurses, and clinical nurse educators having opportunities to offer comments during focus group interviews. After this extensive development process, face validity, but no other psychometric testing, was reported. The tool assesses 12 learning outcomes grouped into four categories: nursing, documentation, caring, and skills and manual handling. These outcomes were chosen based upon required qualifications for RNs in Sweden. The tool outlines standards of achievement for each outcome and criteria for exceeding expectations, meeting expectations, and failing to meet expectations. The tool provides a guide for clinical nurse educators to summatively assess learning outcomes while allowing the freedom to engage in formative assessment of student learning throughout the clinical learning experience. The authors indicate that further testing is needed prior to determination of this tool as a valid and reliable instrument for assessment and evaluation of clinical learning.

Observation

Rubrics and rating tools offer approaches that can aid clinical nurse educators in assessment and evaluation of clinical performance. Other assessment strategies have also been studied. Oermann, Yarbrough, Saewert, Ard, and Charasika (2009b) conducted a survey of clinical grading practices in schools of nursing ($N = 1573$) and found that observation was the predominant clinical evaluation strategy used by clinical nurse educators across all nursing programs. Commonly used strategies for clinical assessment and evaluation are reported in the study by Oermann et al. (2009b) and include written clinical assignments, skills testing, clinical conferences, and student self-assessments. Observational techniques, frequently used by clinical nurse educators, were the predominant clinical evaluation strategy reported by the clinical nurse educators in this study.

There are times when traditional direct observation of students in a clinical site is not feasible or may not even be possible. Clinical nurse educators must then rely on other evaluators, such as preceptors, other means of observation, such as simulation, and additional evaluation strategies to compile evidence of student outcome achievement.

Clinical nurse educators must develop a plan for recording evaluation information and providing student feedback. Anecdotal notes are one such assessment and evaluation strategy to record observations of student performance in the clinical setting. Hall, Daly, and Madigan (2010) detail the use of anecdotal notes by clinical nursing educators as a method of assessment and evaluation. They define anecdotal notes as "a dated, student-specific notation by a clinical nursing faculty member, describing any component of the student's clinical performance" (p. 157). Most clinical nursing faculty report weekly use of anecdotal notes in clinical evaluation (68.8 percent); another 28.1 percent reported the occasional use of notes during the clinical semester. Topics such as medication administration accuracy, patient safety, and professionalism are considered essential in anecdotal note use by clinical nurse educators. Although lack of reliability and validity limits the efficacy of anecdotal notes, they serve as a tool for clinical nurse educators to use to provide supportive data in formative and summative evaluation of clinical performance.

Simulation

Evaluating students in a simulated patient environment is another way clinical nurse educators can assess learner outcome achievement. The use of valid, reliable evaluation tools in simulation is critical. Adamson, Kardong-Edgren, and Willhaus (2013) completed a review of simulation evaluation instruments for the period from 2010 to 2013, updating research from 2010 (Kardong-Edgren, Adamson, & Fitzgerald, 2010). Four instruments were reviewed because of repeated use and reports in the literature: the Sweeny-Clark Simulation Performance Evaluation Tool, the Clinical Simulation Evaluation Tool, the Lasater Clinical Judgment Rubric, and the Creighton Competency Evaluation Instrument (CCEI). The continued use and development of these simulation evaluation tools are an affirmation of Kardong-Edgren et al.'s (2010) insistence on the use and development of tools appropriate for the assessment and evaluation of nursing learners in simulation.

Oermann et al. (2016) conducted a study to determine the likelihood of using a high-stakes simulation experience as a method of evaluating nursing learners' clinical performance. Learners were volunteer nursing students from prelicensure programs across the United States; simulation scenarios were pilot tested at 10 nursing schools and video recorded. A group of experts convened by the National League for Nursing selected four outcomes to evaluate clinical performance: assessment and intervention, nursing judgment, quality and safety, and teamwork and collaboration. The researchers selected the CCEI, which includes 23 skills categorized into four groups relating to four outcomes, for use in this study. Trained evaluators viewed recorded simulation experiences from nine test schools and convened for 3 days to score their assigned videos —each evaluator had 21 to 28 videos to evaluate over 16 hours. The evaluators found that the majority of learners could perform most of the skills on the CCEI. Although several items on the tool resulted in more than 50 percent agreement between evaluators, inconsistencies in interrater reliability occurred for various items, resulting in scoring variations. Further research is needed to understand clinical competence evaluation in simulation by clinical nurse educators.

Objective Structured Clinical Examination

Like traditional simulation, OSCE represents a strategy that clinical nurse educators use to assess and evaluate learners. Clinical nurse educators use OSCEs for formative and summative assessment and the evaluation of clinical performance. Cazzell and Howe (2012) completed a study to determine interrater reliability using a 14-item checklist for a pediatric medication administration OSCE that measured competencies in the affective, psychomotor, and cognitive domains. Two raters evaluated nursing student performance using 207 videotapes of OSCEs. Acceptable interrater reliability was achieved for most items within the psychomotor and cognitive domains of the tool. However, four items within the affective domain obtained inadequate interrater reliability scores. Unfortunately, the reliability of the overall OSCE checklist studied was determined not to be transferable to other checklists with different parameters. The researchers concluded that clinical nurse educators must determine the reliability of each OSCE checklist created due to variability in OSCE setup, competencies or skills assessed, number of evaluators, and method of grading. Clinical nurse educators continue to struggle to find valid and reliable assessment and evaluation strategies.

IDENTIFIED GAPS IN THE LITERATURE

Being an expert clinician does not automatically equate to being an expert assessor or evaluator of student performance. However, to ensure safety and accuracy of clinical practice, it is critical that clinical nurse educators adequately and accurately assess student achievement of learning outcomes and clinical competence. Most textbooks focused on clinical teaching in nursing include entire chapters devoted exclusively to clinical evaluation (Gaberson et al., 2015; O'Connor, 2015; Oermann, 2015), suggesting the critical importance of this topic for clinical nurse educators. Although many assessment and evaluation strategies exist, no one method of evaluation has been found to be used universally that can definitively determine a student's clinical competence. Instead, various assessment and evaluation strategies are available for the clinical nurse educator to use.

The review of the literature indicates a disconnect between the development of clinical evaluation strategies and the evaluation of clinical learning outcomes. Some of the articles reviewed describe how a strategy was used for assessment and evaluation. However, many of the reviewed articles do not report directly on the strategy's impact on learning outcomes. Most articles also lack descriptions of the tool's psychometric properties, leaving the reader unsure of the quality of the assessment approach. It is apparent that more research is needed to guarantee the development of reliable and valid tools.

The changing nature of clinical learning sites, particularly acute care hospitals, has led to changes in clinical learning location. The growing use of simulation as a clinical teaching and learning strategy has created increased interest in the evaluation of this clinical education approach. As clinical learning experiences move from acute care settings to community-based experiences, clinical nurse educators need to consider how to conduct assessment and evaluation in these diverse settings as well. Nurse preceptors, who frequently guide students in these settings, can provide input about student performance for clinical nurse educators. However, preceptors may not have the educational background and training needed for this activity, and faculty may need to consider the impact on assessment and evaluation and then provide appropriate guidance.

Choosing the appropriate assessment and evaluation strategy for the variety of clinical sites is the nurse educator's responsibility. However, in addition to an assortment of clinical sites, the variety of clinical teaching strategies used and the assessment and evaluation techniques available can lead to challenges in selecting the appropriate approach to evaluation. Further, the literature does not clearly distinguish preferred assessment and evaluation techniques for different levels of education. Students enter nursing with diverse backgrounds, educational preparation, and experience, and it is unclear if these factors, as well as differences in educational programs (e.g., first-degree prelicensure, second-degree, accelerated, graduate-level, or other program types), impact clinical assessment and evaluation by clinical nurse educators.

As with many of the other clinical nurse educator competencies, studies reported in the literature were conducted in diverse geographic locations. Many of the reported studies addressing assessment and evaluation were conducted in various international locations. This diversity of clinical education settings suggests the importance, interest, and pervasive concern related to clinical assessment and evaluation. Unfortunately, it is unclear if clinical teaching and evaluation approaches differ across the global community. Diverse models of education (e.g., use of preceptors rather than direct faculty supervision) may impact who evaluates students, what is evaluated, and how and when evaluation is conducted.

PRIORITIES FOR FUTURE RESEARCH

The lack of published best practice and easily transferable, psychometrically sound tools for use in all levels of nursing education has led to variable subjective assessment and evaluation practices among clinical nurse educators. Clinical nurse educators must be able to use assessment and evaluation data to enhance teaching and student learning in the clinical environment. Currently, very little consistent evidence-based research exists to support clinical nurse educators in this area. The following questions reflect priorities for further research:

➤ What are the clinical nurse educator best practices for evaluating clinical learning and ensuring clinical competence of nursing students?

➤ What tools provide valid and reliable assessments of nursing student clinical performance?

➤ How does clinical evaluation of students differ across clinical teaching sites (e.g., simulation laboratory, clinical setting) and clinical locations (e.g., acute care, community health)?

➤ How does clinical evaluation of students differ across nursing program types (e.g., vocational, diploma, associate, baccalaureate, master, doctoral, and pre- and postlicensure)?

➤ How can clinical nurse educators work effectively with clinical preceptors to ensure that proper assessment and evaluation occur during preceptor experiences?

References

Adamson, K. A., Kardong-Edgren, S., & Willhaus, J. (2013). An updated review of published simulation evaluation instruments. *Clinical Simulation in Nursing, 9,* e393–e400. https://doi.org/10.1016/j.ecns.2012.09.004

Bonnel, W. (2016). Clinical performance evaluation. In D. M. Billings & J. A. Halstead

(Eds.), *Teaching in nursing* (5th ed., pp. 443–462). St. Louis, MO: Elsevier.

Cazzell, M., & Howe, C. (2012). Using objective structured clinical evaluation for simulation evaluation: Checklist considerations for interrater reliability. *Clinical Simulation in Nursing, 8*(6), e219–e225. doi:10.1016/j.ecns.2011.10.004

Clark, N. J., Alcala-Van Houten, L., & Perea-Ryan, M. (2010). Transitioning from clinical practice to academia. *Nurse Educator, 35*(3), 105–109. doi:10.1097/NNE.0b013e3181d95069

Dattilo, J., Brewer, M. K., & Streit, L. (2009). Voices of experience: Reflections of nurse educators. *Journal of Continuing Education in Nursing, 40*(8), 367–370. doi:10.3928/00220124-20090723-02

Esmaeili, M., Cheraghi, M. A., Salsali, M., & Ghiyasvandian, S. (2014). Nursing students' expectations regarding effective clinical education: A qualitative study. *International Journal of Nursing Practice, 20*(5), 460–467. doi:10.1111/ijn.12159

Forbes, M. O., Hickey, M. T., & White, J. (2010). Adjunct faculty development: Reported needs and innovative solutions. *Journal of Professional Nursing, 26*(2), 116–124. doi:10.1016/j.profnurs.2009.08.001

Gaberson, K. B., Oermann, M. H., & Shellenbarger, T. (2015). *Clinical teaching strategies in nursing* (4th ed.). New York, NY: Springer.

Girija, K. M. (2012). Effective clinical instructor: A step toward excellence in clinical teaching. *International Journal of Nursing Education, 4*(1), 25–27.

Greiner, A. C., & Knebel, E. (2003). Health professions education: A bridge to quality. Washington DC: National Academies Press.

Hall, M. A., Daly, B. J., & Madigan, E. A. (2010). Use of anecdotal notes by clinical nursing faculty: A descriptive study. *Journal of Nursing Education, 49*(3), 156–159. doi:10.3928/01484834-20090915-3

Hemman, E. A., Gillingham, D., Allison, N., & Adams, R. (2007). Evaluation of a combat medic skills validation test. *Military Medicine, 172*(8), 843–851.

Hewitt, P., & Lewallen, L. (2010). Ready, set, teach! How to transform the clinical nurse expert into the part-time clinical nurse instructor. *The Journal of Continuing Education in Nursing, 41*, 403–407. doi:10.3928/00220124-20100503-10

Holaday, S. D., & Buckley, K. M. (2008). A standardized clinical evaluation tool-kit: Improving nursing education and practice. In M. H. Oermann & K. T. Heinrich (Eds.), *Annual review of nursing education (Vol. 6)*. New York, NY: Springer, 123–149.

Isaacson, J. J., & Stacy, A. S. (2009). Rubrics for clinical evaluation: Objectifying the subjective experience. *Nurse Education in Practice, 9*(2), 134–140. doi:10.1016/j.nepr.2008.10.015

Kardong-Edgren, S., Adamson, K. A., & Fitzgerald, C. (2010). A review of currently published evaluation instruments for human patient simulation. *Clinical Simulation in Nursing, 6*(1), e25–e35. doi:10.1016/j.ecns.2009.08.004

McCarthy, B., & Murphy, S. (2008). Assessing undergraduate nursing students in clinical practice: Do preceptors use assessment strategies? *Nurse Education Today, 28*(3), 301–313. doi:10.1016/j.nedt.2007.06.002

O'Connor, A. B. (2015). *Clinical instruction and evaluation: A teaching resource.* Burlington, MA: Jones & Bartlett.

O'Connor, T., Fealy, G. M., Kelly, M., McGuinness, A. M., & Timmins, F. (2009). An evaluation of a collaborative approach to the assessment of competence among nursing students of three universities in Ireland. *Nurse Education Today, 29*(5), 493–499. doi:10.1016/j.nedt.2008.11.014

Oermann, M. H. (2015). *Teaching in nursing and role of the educator: The complete guide to best practice in teaching, evaluation, and curriculum development.* New York, NY: Springer.

Oermann, M. H., & Gaberson, K. B. (2017). *Evaluation and testing in nursing education* (5th ed.). New York, NY: Springer.

Oermann, M. H., Kardong-Edgren, S., & Rizzolo, M. A. (2016). Towards an evidence-based methodology for high-stakes evaluation of nursing students' clinical performance using simulation. *Teaching and Learning in Nursing, 11*(4), 133–137. doi:10.1016/j.teln.2016.04.001

Oermann, M. H., Saewert, K. J., Charasika, M., & Yarbrough, S. S. (2009a). Assessment and grading practices in schools of nursing: National survey findings part I. *Nursing Education Perspectives, 30*(5), 274–278.

Oermann, M. H., Yarbrough, S. S., Saewert, K. J., Ard, N., & Charasika, M. (2009b). Clinical evaluation and grading practices in schools of nursing: National survey findings part II. *Nursing Education Perspectives, 30*(6), 352–357.

Prion, S. K., Gilbert, G. E., Adamson, K. A., Kardong-Edgren, S., & Quint, S. (2017). Development and testing of the Quint Leveled Clinical Competency Tool. *Clinical Simulation in Nursing, 13*(3), 106–115. doi:10.1016/j.ecns.2016.10.008

Selim, A. A., Ramadan, F. H., El-Gueneidy, M. M., & Gaafer, M. M. (2012). Using objective structured clinical examination (OSCE) in undergraduate psychiatric nursing education: Is it reliable and valid? *Nurse Education Today, 32*(3), 283–288. doi:10.1016/j/nedt.2011.04.006

Skúladóttir, H., & Svavarsdóttir, M. H. (2016). Development and validation of a Clinical Assessment Tool for Nursing

Education (CAT-NE). *Nurse Education in Practice, 20*(2016), 31–38. doi:10.1016/j.nepr.2016.06.008

Stevens, L., & Mattsson, J. Y. (2016). Development of an individual assessment instrument for critical care nursing students. *Journal of Nursing Education and Practice, 7*(2), 1–13. doi:10.5430/jnep.v7n2p54

Sullivan, D. T. (2016). An introduction to curriculum development. In D. M. Billings & J. A. Halstead (Eds.), *Teaching in nursing: A guide for faculty* (5th ed., pp. 89–117). St. Louis, MO: Elsevier.

Tanner, C. A. (2006). Thinking like a nurse: A research-based model of clinical judgment in nursing. *Journal of Nursing Education, 45*(6), 204–211. doi:10.1046/j.1365-2648.2003.02921.x

Ulfvarson, J., & Oxelmark, L. (2012). Developing an assessment tool for intended learning outcomes in clinical practice for nursing students. *Nurse Education Today, 32*(6), 703–708. doi:10.1016/j.nedt.2011.09.010

Wu, X. V., Enskär, K., Lee, C. C. S., & Wang, W. (2015). A systematic review of clinical assessment for undergraduate nursing students. *Nurse Education Today, 35*(2), 347–359. doi:10/1016/j.nedt.2014.11.016